MASTERING HORMONES AND HEALTH FOR WOMEN 35+

Learn to Take Charge of your Health Using Scientific Facts and the Wisdom of your Intuition

DR. GEORGINA HALE, MD, Ph.D.

Mastering Hormones and Health for Women 35+
Learn to Take Charge of your Health Using Scientific Facts and the
Wisdom of your Intuition

Published by Hale Health Medicine

ISBN: 978-1-7638998-0-3
        978-1-7638998-1-0 (paperback)
        978-1-7638998-2-7 (ebook)

NATIONAL LIBRARY OF AUSTRALIA

A catalogue record for this
book is available from the
National Library of Australia

Typeset by Midland Typesetters, Australia
Printed by IngramSpark

Contents

Section One

The Basics: How your reproductive body works   1

Section Two

Your Zone: Your hormones and symptoms explained   35

Section Three

The Solutions 99

Is this book for you?

- Are you 35 or older and want meaningful information about how your body and hormones might be changing?
- Are your periods causing you pain or discomfort when they didn't before?
- Are you feeling more abdominal discomfort and/or feeling more bloated?
- Are you feeling sluggish or 'heavy' and find it hard to shift the weight around your midriff?
- Are you having trouble falling asleep or staying asleep at night?
- Are you getting more headaches and/or experiencing forgetfulness and foggy thinking?
- Do you get easily overwhelmed, emotional or irritable in response to things that in the past were no big deal?
- Has your libido vanished?
- Are you getting more urinary tract infections than you used to?
- Do you need to take prescription medications to help you function?
- Are you willing to take the steps needed to understand your body and learn what you can do yourself to feel good again?

If you have answered YES to any of these, this book is likely a good one for you.

About the Author

Dr. Georgina Hale is an Australian medical specialist in internal medicine and infectious diseases. Following her extensive medical specialist training, Dr. Hale completed a Ph.D. in midlife women's reproductive endocrinology (hormones) at the University of Sydney. She also has a diploma in public health, and has studied functional medicine since 2014, gaining a certification with the Institute of Functional Medicine in 2016. This book is Dr. Hale's first publication where she presents her Ph.D. research findings in an easy-to-understand format for the everyday woman. She illustrates the importance of understanding her unique Ph.D. findings and presents them along with other important up-to-date women's health information for midlife and menopausal women.

Dr. Hale's Ph.D. findings were indeed unique. She herself designed and carried out the study which involved performing regular blood hormone measurements in women aged 45 to 55 while tracking their symptoms and menstrual blood flow. Her small but important study contributed greatly to the scientific literature and deepened our understanding of the hormonal changes at midlife and during the transition to menopause. She cites Professors Claude L. Hughes and Ian S. Fraser as important mentors in helping her mastermind the study design that allowed for these novel results. Professors Henry Burger in Melbourne and Noel Bairey Merz in Los Angeles were also very important in supporting her in the early days of creating the study and throughout. Dr. Hale is especially thankful to the Australasian Menopause Society who funded and made her research possible at the University of Sydney. Her novel research led to her being awarded the American Menopause Society's Chilcott Research award in 2008.

Following her Ph.D., Dr. Hale has continued to expand her internal medicine expertise and knowledge, exploring ways to improve patient care and outcomes. The unique combination of novel insights from her research and her lengthy experience in both conventional and functional medicine, allows her to listen to patients in a way which is far beyond the disease-drug model that she initially trained in. In this way, she along with other forward-thinking clinical practitioners are creating a brighter future for individualized patient care in both women's health and patient care in general.

Here is a small selection of her Ph.D. related peer reviewed publications:

Hale, G.E. and H.G. Burger, *Hormonal changes and biomarkers in late reproductive age, menopausal transition and menopause.* Best Practice & Research in Clinical Obstetrics & Gynaecology, 2009. **23**(1): p. 7-23

Hale, G.E., et al., *Atypical estradiol secretion and ovulation patterns caused by luteal out-of-phase (LOOP) events underlying irregular ovulatory menstrual cycles in the menopausal transition.* Menopause, 2009. **16**(1): p. 50-9

Hale, G.E., C.L. Hughes, and J.M. Cline, *Clinical review 139 - Endometrial cancer: Hormonal factors, the perimenopausal "window of risk," and isoflavones [Review].* Journal of Clinical Endocrinology & Metabolism, 2002. **87**(1): p. 3-15

Hale, G.E., et al., *Quantitative measurements of menstrual blood loss in ovulatory and anovulatory cycles in middle- and late-reproductive age and the menopausal transition.* Obstetrics & Gynecology, 2010. **115**(2 Pt 1): p. 249-56

Hale, G.E., et al., *Endocrine features of menstrual cycles in middle and late reproductive age and the menopausal transition classified according to the Staging of Reproductive Aging Workshop (STRAW) staging system.* Journal of Clinical Endocrinology & Metabolism, 2007. **92**(8): p. 3060-7

From Dr. Hale to You the reader

My motivation for writing this book was to have you become skilled and confident at navigating your way through midlife: your late thirties, forties, and fifties. Midlife can be a tumultuous time for women, with many experiencing unpredictable and heavy bleeding, unexplained weight gain, feelings of overwhelm, disturbed sleep, low libido, headaches, and more. These experiences result from more extreme and erratic hormonal ups and downs that are part of what many of us refer to as the 'hormonal storm'. Midlife is like the *storm* before the *calm* of menopause when the monthly hormonal ups and downs are winding down. The 'hormonal storm' is a reflection of the aging of our reproductive system, with our ovaries being the focus of this aging process.

Through Sections One, Two and Three, I will cover the **What's**, the **Why's**, and the **To-Do's**. The Section One **What's** are about the body and brain components of your reproductive system and the typical changes that occur from about age 35. The Section Two **Why's** are about the wide range of symptoms that can occur as a result of this reproductive aging. By monitoring the changes in your menstrual cycle and 'tuning into' your body's symptoms, you can learn how to determine where you are at in terms of your reproductive aging. This involves determining which **Reproductive Zone** you are in, and I will explain this below. The Section Three **To-Do's** concern the medical, diet and lifestyle strategies unique to each Zone. These strategies can be uniquely tailored to you because they are based on your personal **Reproductive Zone**. You can implement these strategies on your own or in collaboration with a healthcare provider.

Know your reproductive Zone: The key to navigating through your hormonal journey

If it is not already obvious, one of the main aims I had in writing this book was to bring the science to you, the everyday woman. Much work has been done by the research community to devise ways to understand and characterize the changes that occur with reproductive aging. Indeed, I was part of a group of experts and researchers who helped create the Stages of Reproductive Aging system or 'STRAW' system. I used this scientific system to plan, carry out and publish data from my Ph.D. research study. My familiarity with this STRAW system helped me devise a user-friendly version for the purposes of this book. I refer to this 'stepped down' version of the STRAW system as the **Reproductive Zones**. I explain the Reproductive Zones in detail in **Section One**, and then in **Section Two**, I explain how you can determine your own Zone by tracking your menstrual cycle and/ or tuning into your body's symptoms. Once you have identified the Zone that you are currently in, you can read the **To-Do's** in **Section Three**, knowing which dietary, lifestyle and other strategy to focus on. Being familiar with your unique hormone/body characteristics in addition to your Zone will also help you develop the skills to maintain optimal health well into the future.

As you may have guessed, Zone 1, Zone 2, Zone 3 and Zone 4 represent the Zones that you progress through from your mid to late-30s to menopause. It makes sense therefore, that if you are in Zone 1 now, over time you will progress through the Zones to Zone 4. All of us experience Zone 1 and Zone 4, but not everyone experiences the in-between zones, Zone 2 and Zone 3. Some women skip Zone 2 and/or Zone 3. This will make more sense when I explain the Zones in detail in Section One.

Functional and conventional medicine: An important combination for women

Prior to starting my Ph.D. research into women's hormones, I was not aware of the myriad of hormonal changes that could occur before menopause, and, like many other medical doctors, I only knew about 'the menopause', and its associated hot flushes, and the estrogen-containing hormone medications. One of the most important things I realized through the preparation and completion of my Ph.D. was the huge gap in medical knowledge surrounding the changes in midlife women's hormones prior to menopause. And while one could argue that these gaps didn't matter, most women start to get worrisome symptoms well before menopause. These symptoms include heavy bleeding, sore breasts, low mood, emotional upheaval, memory deficits, bloating, and midriff weight gain. I realized that these typical midlife symptoms were, more likely than not, a result of changes in hormones. Although my Ph.D. didn't 'prove' that midlife women's symptoms were caused by hormonal changes, my Ph.D. certainly provided clarity about the wide variety of hormonal and symptom changes that can occur. However it wasn't until I studied functional medicine, that I acquired more understanding about why many midlife women have symptoms as hormones change with reproductive aging. It certainly isn't simply due to a loss of hormones, as one could expect after reaching menopause.

My conventional specialist medical practice had largely confined me to diagnosing and treating diseases. So, if a woman presented with symptoms that didn't indicate a recognized disease, my therapeutic approach was often limited to symptom-relief medications. My conventional training didn't give me the expertise to work through the reasons why her symptoms may be occurring, or how she could alleviate them through addressing some of the underlying causes unique to her. For example, if a forty-year-old woman came to my practice with sleep disturbance, increased irritability, midriff weight gain, and heavy bleeding, the only approach I knew with conventional medicine was to offer prescription medication such as a sleeping pill, an analgesic, an antidepressant, or even the birth control pill. I simply wouldn't have had the knowledge to explain to her why she might be experiencing these symptoms in the first place.

Not only did the functional medicine training allow me to give my patients an understanding of their symptoms and likely related hormone changes, but it also gave me expertise in devising effective diet and lifestyle strategies that they could use to help reduce symptoms. For example, in some women, breast soreness, midriff weight gain, or heavy bleeding can be an indicators of rising estrogen levels. The ensuing consultation, therefore, may involve an explanation of her symptoms and some strategies to help her body process her own estrogen and other hormones more effectively. The consultation would also involve talking about how stress, poor diet, and poor gut health can trigger rising estrogen levels and adversely affect her symptoms and overall future health. Simply put, understanding how best to improve your own health today will greatly reduce the burden and adverse consequences of any health issues tomorrow.

Foreword

Well, dear reader, thank you for taking the time to read this wee bit of perspective! Yes, you are indeed continuing your journey through your unique life, but now you will have the cogent and comprehensible expertise of Dr. Georgina Hale at hand, as together you may proceed with "Mastering Hormones and Health for Women 35+"!

I know full well that continuation of this journey of yours will be more fulfilling and reassuring than you can presently imagine. Georgina and I have been colleagues for the last quarter of a century(!), and I know that along with her intrinsic wisdom and respect for individual sensibilities, her scientific and clinical expertise is eloquently translated into erudite but understandable explanations throughout the following book. Without any element of "talking down to you," Dr. Hale communicates the complex reproductive endocrinology of midlife women in a conversational but scientifically rigorous manner that respects the intuition that each woman possesses as an important part of her internal skillset for understanding, accepting, and adapting to the changes that occur across this phase of her lifespan.

In her book, Dr. Hale has kindly referenced several of us older colleagues who worked with her in the past as she conducted her research projects to better understand the hormonal changes that occur in women from their mid-30s onwards in life. However, she deserves the lioness's share of credit for inspiring and leading the research completed in those past years. Now from both scientific and caregiver perspectives, she is adding to that legacy with this book to serve as the important presentation of those clarifying insights that will be accessible to all of you who are, after all, living the experiences she investigated. Her synthesis relies on the scientific and medical facts to provide a coherent description of the reproductive endocrinology of midlife women that will be informative to all readers, no matter whether they are members of the public at large, healthcare providers, or even intensely invested biomedical investigators (like me)!

One source of immense pride for those of us who mentor junior colleagues in biomedical research is to see them become our professional peers, and then in turn, the intellectual leaders who begin to teach all of us. As I was reading this book from cover to cover, I was endlessly smiling with the clarity of the conversation that I felt Georgina was having with me. Her insightful blend of scientific data, medical expertise, and respect for each person's intuition showed me a way to better communicate with my own patients into the future. Thank you, Dr. Hale for this new mentoring of me! I'm confident that other experienced healthcare professionals will feel the same way after they read this book.

So, if you're a woman who is 35 or 45 or 55 years old or more, or someone who cares deeply for that woman, then finally there is this book for you! If you are ready to have a sustained informative conversation with that most knowledgeable non-judgmental friend in your life, who will always respect your individuality and understand your reticence to express some of your concerns, then now that person for you can be Dr. Georgina Hale via this outstanding book.

Durham, North Carolina, USA 10 January 2025
Claude Hughes, M.D., Ph.D.
Consulting Professor
Reproductive Endocrinology and Infertility
Department of Obstetrics & Gynecology
Duke University Medical Center

The Basics:

How your reproductive body works

This section of the book contains the 'nitty-gritty' nuts and bolts information about your hormones and your body during the 15 or so years prior to menopause, and when menopause arrives.

Here are some of the topics covered in this section:

- What your reproductive body and reproductive hormones are.
- How your brain and your ovaries communicate with each other to produce the reproductive hormones.
- How your hormones create your menstrual cycle and how the process is like a kind of 'stage play', with the brain being the main director.
- What makes your ovary and its *ovarian follicles* so special and how they are key to what happens at midlife.
- How your Reproductive Zone tells you where you are at in terms of your current 'stage' of reproductive aging.
- What happens to hormones in each Reproductive Zone and how you can approach hormone testing.
- Understanding what is referred to as 'estrogen dominance'.
- Understanding what is often referred to as 'hormone imbalance' and what it may mean for you.

Your reproductive body

Your reproductive body is made up of the:

- ovaries
- uterus and fallopian tubes
- pituitary gland and hypothalamus in the brain.

The ovaries contain your female germ cells or eggs, also called ova (single is *ovum*). In research and science literature, they are usually referred to as *ovarian follicles*. Your ovaries and your ovarian follicles determine what kind of hormonal changes you will experience at midlife. I explain this later in this section. The uterus and fallopian tubes, next to the ovary, are primarily for conception and pregnancy, and any hormones produced by them are primarily to coordinate fertility and pregnancy. The pituitary gland and hypothalamus within the brain produce specific hormones that 'talk to' the ovary and coordinate ovarian follicle activity to orchestrate fertility and the menstrual cycle. The communication system between the brain and ovary is highly coordinated and complex. It is also inherently intelligent and self-adjusting and is influenced by all manner of activities going on within your body and in your surrounding environment. We all know as menstrual-cycling women that outside influences or illness can change *when* we get a period, how much we bleed, how much pain or discomfort we have, how tense we feel during the days leading up to it, and how much it affects our daily lives each month.

The creation of your menstrual cycle: A 'stage play'

Understanding new and complex concepts can be easier if we use analogies. I invite you to think of your reproductive system as a 'stage play'. The director of this play being the hypothalamus, the assistant director being the pituitary, the ovary being the supplier of your hormones that are the necessary stage props and actresses in the stage play. Our menstrual cycle, the menstrual period and all the symptoms associated with this are the stage play itself.

The hormones in your reproductive stage play:

GnRH: gonadotropin-releasing hormone is produced in the hypothalamus and controls hormone production from the pituitary gland, the ovary, and ovarian follicles. Understandably, GnRH is often referred to as the 'master hormone'.

FSH: follicle-stimulating hormone is produced in the pituitary gland and stimulates the growth and activity of the ovarian follicles and ovarian hormone production.

LH: luteinizing hormone is produced in the pituitary gland and coordinates the process of ovulation whereby an egg is expelled each month in preparation for a pregnancy.

Inhibin B (INHB): this hormone is named 'inhibin' because it 'inhibits' the production of FSH from the pituitary gland. INHB levels fall when the number of ovarian follicles falls (this is what occurs at midlife), and the *fall* in INHB leads to a *rise* in FSH. More on this 'negative feedback' mechanism later.

Estrogen is one of the *steroid* or *sex* hormones produced in the ovary. It rises and falls in the blood circulation in a highly coordinated manner to create the menstrual cycle. It is responsible for breast development in puberty and during breast feeding and supports the development of the other physical body changes during puberty such as pubic hair and subcutaneous fat stores. Estrogen also plays a role outside of the reproductive system, including in blood vessel function, blood fat/lipid regulation, skin and collagen elasticity, mood, and bone strength.

Progesterone is another *steroid* or *sex* hormone and like estrogen is produced in the ovary. It is different in that it is produced by a specialized 'pocket' of follicular cells that is left behind in the ovary after ovulation, called the *corpus luteum*. This is why progesterone is only produced in high amounts after ovulation, and why the second half of the menstrual cycle is called the *luteal* phase. It is mainly the rapid fall in progesterone levels at the end of the luteal phase (if pregnancy doesn't occur) that triggers menstrual bleeding. Progesterone is also produced outside of the ovary, but only in very small amounts by the adrenal glands and the brain. As a circulating bloodstream hormone, it plays many roles in the body including in water balance, mood, cognitive function, immunity, inflammation, bone health, and the body's energy processes (mitochondria function).

Testosterone is another *steroid* or *sex* hormone and like estrogen and progesterone is produced in the ovary. Testosterone does not play as key a role in creating the menstrual cycle as estrogen and progesterone but likely plays a role in the follicle maturing process and expulsion, brain and nerve function, mood, bone health, and the body's energy processes.

Table 1: The chain of command in your reproductive stage play

The Reproductive Stage Play		
Stage play member	**Hormone**	**Place in body where the hormone is made**
Director	GnRH	Hypothalamus in the brain
Assistant director	FSH and LH	Pituitary in the brain
Stage managers	The inhibins including INHB B	Ovaries
Actresses	Steroid hormones including estrogen, progesterone and testosterone	Ovarian follicles and corpus luteum
The reproductive stage play you experience includes your menstrual cycle, menstrual bleeding, and any symptoms you may feel as a result		

How your hormones create your menstrual cycle

Estrogen and progesterone are the two main hormones that create your menstrual cycle, with testosterone playing a minor role in the growth and release of the ovum.

Figure 1: Follicles, ovulation, and the menstrual cycle

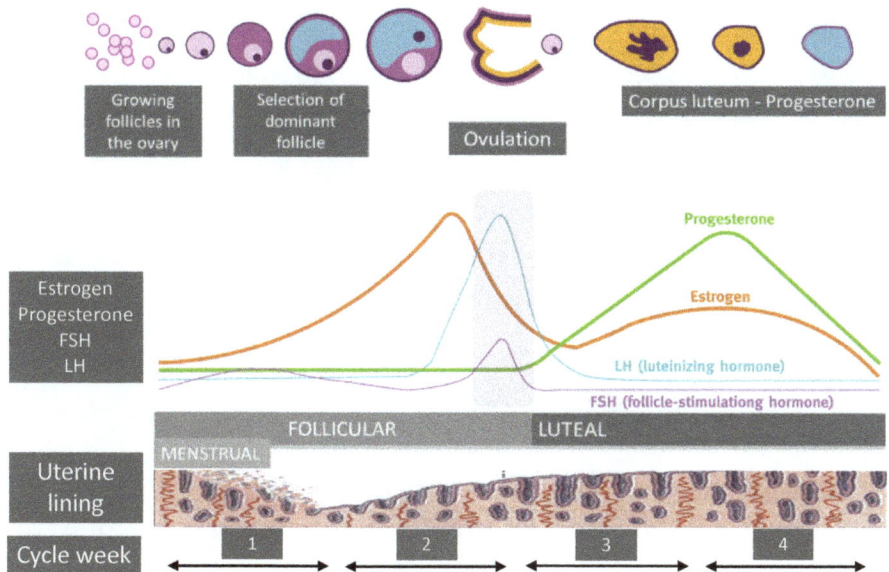

Figure 1 depicts a healthy 28-day menstrual cycle divided into four one-week blocks, with week 1 and 2 making up the *follicular* phase and weeks 3 and 4 making up the *luteal* phase. The *menstrual* phase is 3-7 days long and is considered part of the early follicular phase. As the name implies, the follicular phase is when the ovarian follicles in the ovary start growing and maturing in readiness to be expelled at ovulation. They grow and mature in response to rising estrogen levels. Notice in the figure how estrogen levels rise to peak during the follicular phase, then fall at midcycle after ovulation when an ovum is expelled. Estrogen levels then rise again during the luteal phase. The luteal phase is also when progesterone levels rise (weeks 3 and 4). As I mentioned before, progesterone is made and released by the pocket of cells called the *corpus luteum* which forms after an ovum is expelled at ovulation. The growth of the ovarian follicle, ovulation and the formation of the corpus luteum after mid-cycle is depicted at the top of the figure.

At the bottom of the figure, you can see a drawing of the lining of the uterus or *endometrium*. Notice how the endometrium falls away during the first five or so days of the menstrual cycle when menstrual bleeding occurs. Notice the endometrium starts to build up after again at the end of the menstrual phase in response to rising estrogen. After ovulation, the endometrium responds to the rise in progesterone, undergoing dramatic changes in blood vessels and glands in readiness to receive a fertilized ovum and to support the growth of a new life. These dramatic changes are referred to as *decidualization* of the endometrium. If a pregnancy doesn't occur, levels of estrogen and progesterone rapidly fall. It is the rapid fall in the level of progesterone in particular, that triggers a breakdown of the decidualized endometrium, and this is the menstrual bleed.

Your brain as the director of your reproductive stage play

The hypothalamus is like the director of your reproductive stage play and the pituitary is the assistant director. Both are very tiny structures that lie in the center of your brain. The director-hypothalamus kick starts the stage play in most women about once a month on a cyclical basis when no pregnancy occurs. Through its complex hormone-sensing abilities, the director-hypothalamus detects when a pregnancy hasn't occurred and it 'puts the call out' for another stage play to begin (to try for another pregnancy). It does this by producing the GnRH hormone, which travels down a short distance to the pituitary gland, situated immediately under the hypothalamus. The GnRH 'directs' the assistant director, pituitary to start producing its hormone, FSH.

FSH travels in the blood system to the ovary and is detected by the ovarian follicles. This is the ovarian follicles' signal to start developing an ovum within an ovarian follicle in readiness to expel one again at ovulation. The ovarian follicles in turn start producing the sex hormones that become the actresses in the stage play. The technical name for this stage play is the *'hypothalamo-pituitary-ovarian axis* or *feedback cycle'*. It is called a 'feedback' cycle because of the complex way these hormones 'feed' messages back and forward to coordinate the whole. You can see an illustration of this feedback sequence in **Figure 2**. The LH produced by the pituitary works a little differently to FSH. Instead of *causing* a rise in estrogen as FSH does, it rises *in*

Figure 2: How the brain, hypothalamus, pituitary, ovary, and uterus connect

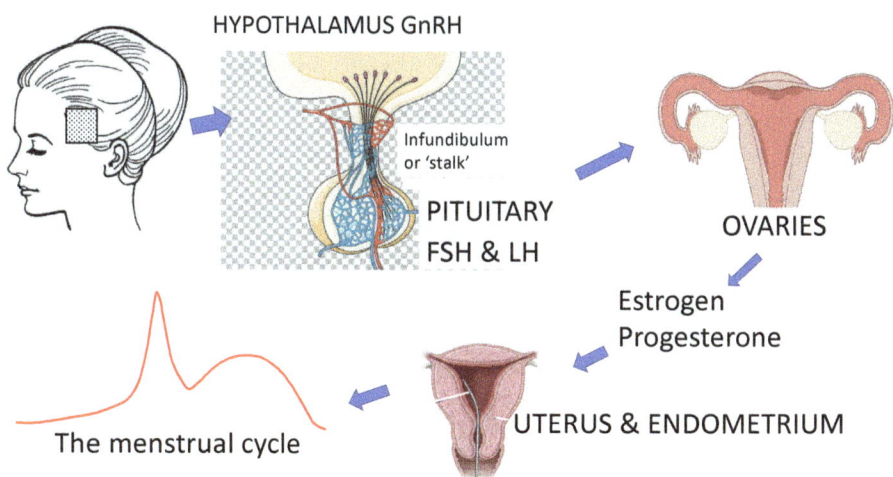

HYPOTHALAMUS GnRH

Infundibulum or 'stalk'

PITUITARY FSH & LH

OVARIES

Estrogen Progesterone

UTERUS & ENDOMETRIUM

The menstrual cycle

response to estrogen. In fact, it is the rapid rise in estrogen in the middle of cycle that signals the pituitary to release LH. This is referred to as the 'mid-cycle LH peak'. The LH peak is instrumental in triggering ovulation, the release of a mature ovum at midcycle.

The changes in the stage play at midlife: The ovary has the final say

One of the many mysteries of reproduction lies in the ovary and the activity of the ovarian follicles. Even though only one or two ova are released at midcycle every month, it is estimated that at least *thirty* ovarian follicles undergo the preparation process to release an ovum each month. Once these thirty or more ovarian follicles have started this preparation and growth process, they cannot reverse it. This irreversible process results in the loss of each of these thirty or so developing follicles, even though only one or two are expelled at ovulation. The ones that are not expelled stay in the ovary, shrink then disappear. The scientific term for this is 'follicular atresia'. This is one of the reasons we lose so many ovarian follicles during our short 35-40-year reproductive life! **Figure 3** shows how ovarian follicles develop and grow each month. There are obviously *far* fewer ovarian follicles depicted in the illustration that what actually develop in an ovary every month.

Figure 3: The ovary and its follicles

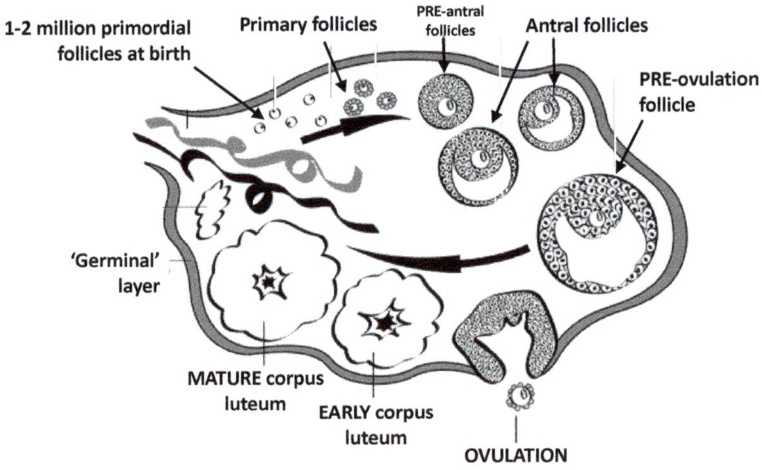

Why do we lose our ovarian follicles?

By the time a woman reaches midlife, there is a dramatic reduction in the number of ovarian follicles compared to what exists at puberty. After at least 30 years of menstrual cycles, the process of follicle atresia has markedly reduced the number of ovarian follicles. Research from my own study and others indicates that the decline in ovarian follicles leads to a decline in the production of INHB. This fall in INHB leads to a rise in FSH. This rise in FSH, in turn, likely accelerates the process of follicle development, then atresia and can, in some women, lead to erratic hormone levels and hormonal symptoms. The initial rise in FSH on blood hormone testing is one of the earliest detectable indicators of midlife and perimenopause. **Figure 4** illustrates a model of how ovarian follicles are lost as the ovaries age.[1]

Figure 4: Loss of ovarian follicles with age

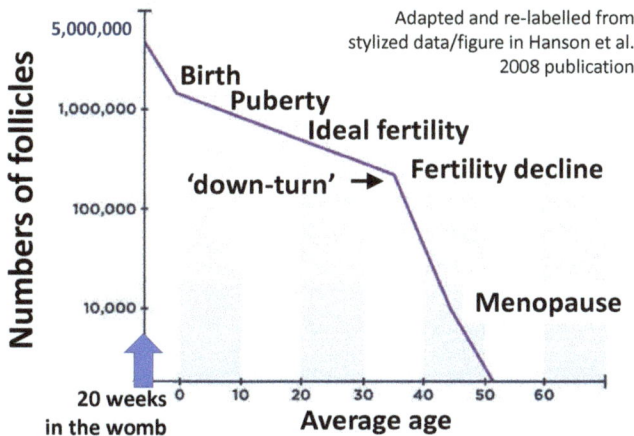

You can see that the number of ovarian follicles actually drops before we are born. In fact, by the time we are a 20-*week*-old unborn female child, we are storing up to *five million follicles* in our ovaries. After this 20-week point as an unborn female child, we don't produce any more ovarian follicles.[2] That's it. Moreover, by the time we are born, we've already lost about *two-thirds* of our ovarian follicles, with the count being down to about half to one million follicles.[3]

As mentioned previously, at least 30 ovarian follicles develop and grow each month, with only 1 or 2 follicles reaching the maturity required to be expelled at ovulation. This would lead to the loss of around 20,000 follicles between puberty and menopause. This is far less than the actual numbers that are lost during this time. It turns out that 2-3 groups of follicles grow and develop each month in what are termed 'follicular waves'.[4] But again, this would still only account for around 60,000 lost follicles over a reproductive lifetime.

This remains a mystery, as does the reason why only around 0.02% of our ovarian follicles go through the maturing process to produce an ovulation. Some researchers have called the loss of ovarian follicles prior to any development 'autophagy'.[5] This process refers to the normal, regulated body mechanism that removes unnecessary or dysfunctional components.[6] One wonders why so many of our follicles are considered 'unnecessary' or 'dysfunctional', but it may have something to do with normal follicle wear and tear. Follicles can be damaged through various mechanisms, including excess inflammation,[7] stress, illness, autoimmunity, cancer, chemotherapy,[8] ovarian surgery, and possibly even our modern-day pollution and/or electro-magnetic radiation exposure.[9]

Why do we lose ovarian follicles at an even higher rate at midlife?
Figure 4 shows another important feature. It shows the *accelerated* loss of follicles at midlife. Some authors have referred to the time when follicle loss accelerates as the 'down-turn'. Notably, this point has also been shown to correspond with a marked reduction in fertility.[10, 11] The cause for this accelerated follicle loss at midlife is not known, but it likely has something to do with rising FSH levels which has the effect of stimulating more follicles to grow. If more follicles are stimulated to grow, more follicles can be lost through atresia. The aging process itself may also be a factor, because over time, the genetic material stored in the follicles can be damaged. If genetic material in the follicles is damaged, the follicle is more likely to be lost through atresia.

Key points about our ovarian follicles as we age:

- In a 20-week female unborn child, the ovaries contain up to 5 million ovarian follicles; at birth, only one half to one million remain.
- More than 99% of ovarian follicles are lost to atresia or autophagy.
- By menopause, there are only 500-1,000 remaining ovarian follicles in the ovary.
- During the menstrual cycle each month, at least 2 groups of follicles start to grow and develop a mature ovum in readiness for ovulation. However, only one or two follicles a month get to produce an ovum that will ovulate.
- We lose follicles more rapidly by our late 30s and 40s.
- The accelerated loss of ovarian follicles at midlife corresponds with a fall in fertility.

Learning your Reproductive 'Zone'

As previously stated in the introduction pages, I created the **Reproductive Zone system** to help you determine where you are at in terms of your reproductive aging. By knowing your 'Zone', you are better placed to understand your hormones, your symptoms and what you can do about them. The Zones start at Zone 1, at the beginning of midlife, and end at Zone 4 at the onset of menopause. The terms I have used in the Zone system include *late reproductive age, early perimenopause, late perimenopause* and *menopause*.

The Reproductive Zones are based on the **S**tages of **R**eproductive **A**ging **W**orkshop or STRAW System. The STRAW system was first created by a group of women's health experts in 2001 and was then updated in 2010.[12, 13] I was one of a group of experts at the meeting in 2010 who discussed the updates. The 2010 version of this system can be found in **Appendix I** and is called **STRAW+10**. Please take a look if you're interested, but it is by no means a 'must do'.

The Zones correspond to the STRAW stages as follows:
- Zone 1 = late reproductive age = STRAW Stage -3a and -3b
- Zone 2 = early perimenopause = STRAW Stage -2
- Zone 3 = late perimenopause = STRAW stage -1
- Zone 4 = menopause = STRAW Stage +1a and +1b.

Because determining your Zone requires a functioning menstrual cycle, you can't easily determine your Zone if you have had your uterus removed (hysterectomy). However, you can approximate your Zone by reading the following section in which I explain some of the more common symptoms linked to each of the four Zones. You may also have to *approximate* your Zone if you have had longstanding irregular cycles or have other medical reasons for interrupted menstrual cycles.

Zone 1

Late reproductive age

In Zone 1, you are likely to be at least 35 years old. You may or may not have started experiencing *subtle* changes in your usual regular menstrual cycles.

Typical but subtle changes in menstrual cycle and hormones in Zone 1 include:

- shortening of menstrual cycle length from an average of 27-29 to 25-27 days
- rise in FSH usually only detectable if measured at the beginning of the cycle
- rise in estrogen throughout the cycle but not usually detectable on blood hormone testing
- fall in progesterone during the luteal phase but not usually detectable on blood hormone testing.

These changes in Zone 1 are likely to be a result of a fall in your Inhibin B (INHB). In my study and other studies, a fall in INHB has been observed to be the first detectable hormonal change in late reproductive age. This hormone, however, is only measured in the research setting. The fall in INHB leads to a rise in FSH, and this rise may or may not be detected in blood samples during the first 2-7 days of a menstrual cycle. The rise in FSH in turn likely leads to an accelerated loss of ovarian follicles.

Many researchers and clinicians will dispute that estrogen elevations occur in Zone 1, but this has been demonstrated in a number of small studies, including my own.[12, 14] In addition, the slight elevations in FSH and estrogen seem to contribute to the early ovulation and shorter menstrual cycles observed in Zone 1.[15, 16] The slight fall in progesterone in Zone 1 is also often disputed because the detailed blood hormone studies that are needed to fully investigate this are lacking. Slight falls in progesterone were seen in my detailed study but not in another similar study.[12, 17] Progesterone levels may become less consistent with reproductive aging due to a number of factors, including a rise in both FSH and estrogen and a reduced quality of ovarian follicles and thus reduced quality of the corpus luteum.

Although the hormonal and menstrual changes in Zone 1 can be subtle, this is often when women start to experience symptoms. Research into midlife symptoms has begun but to date, only descriptive studies of self-reported symptoms have been published.[18] Thus, symptoms in this Zone are usually considered to be unrelated to changes in hormones. I believe, however, that symptoms in this Zone may indeed result from the hormonal changes occurring and that when they occur, they represent an ideal opportunity for women to understand their bodies and learn how to self-manage health issues. I believe that a women's understanding of her body in Zone 1 allows her to have a better experience through to menopause and to enjoy optimal health in future.

Jess: One of my Zone 1 patients

Jess aged 42, came to see me with sleep disturbance, worsening headaches, mid-cycle pelvic pain, midriff weight gain, increased breast size, and feeling extremely irritable with colleagues at work. She even found herself snapping at her husband, which was very unusual for her. Jess consulted her family doctor and was sure that they would find something wrong. She had become increasingly concerned about early menopause and cancer in her ovaries.

Her doctor ran a series of tests to check her blood count, kidneys, liver, thyroid, iodine levels, hormone levels, and iron levels. To Jess's surprise, she was told everything was fine and that she was 'not starting menopause' yet. Jess was prescribed *an antidepressant and a sleep medication*, and a subsequent check-up appointment was made before Jess departed the office.

I will discuss the series of testing that Jess's doctor would have ordered in **Section Three**, and why Jess's hormone changes were not evident to her doctor. If Jess's complaints were not due to 'menopause', could they still have been due to a change in her hormones? I believe they could. If you have symptoms similar to Jess, please know that just because your medical tests look normal, subtle changes in your hormones may still explain your symptoms. Jess told me that after seeing her doctor, she felt depressed about her outbursts and other symptoms because there didn't seem to be an explanation. She also didn't feel depressed, so she was uncertain as to whether she wanted to try the antidepressant medication. She felt somewhat disempowered, but she did have the courage to ask her doctor to get a referral to come and see me.

Would Jess have felt more empowered if she had understood why and what she could do about her outbursts and her other bothersome symptoms? Probably, yes. Wouldn't she then have been able to create more joy in her life and other people's lives? I'd say absolutely yes. When Jess came to me for an opinion, I told her that although her tests results were showing everything was in the 'normal range', changes in her hormones were still likely to be contributing to her symptoms. I explained that her estrogen levels could be on the rise and that her ovulatory cycles may have started to falter in terms of producing the usual amounts of progesterone. And, yes, although hormonal changes are subtle in Zone 1 and challenging to capture on testing, I assured her that women often seem to 'feel' these changes.

What I wanted Jess to understand was that even though Zone 1 hormone changes are usually subtle, they are truly happening, and the symptoms they may be causing are manageable. I told her that her symptoms represented a perfect opportunity to understand what was going on in her body and that a personalized health management strategy could not only help alleviate her symptoms but also put her in a better place in terms of her current and future health. These strategies and others are discussed in **Section Three**.

Fertility in Zone 1

Some readers may be wondering whether they can still fall pregnant in Zone 1. The answer is yes, and contraception remains a necessary consideration for sexually active couples. The chances of falling pregnant are, however, greatly reduced compared to earlier in life. A successful pregnancy depends on both the number and quality of ovarian follicles in the ovary. The number of ovarian follicles can be estimated by measuring levels of anti-Müllerian hormone or **AMH** in the blood. Fertility specialists use AMH levels to help estimate the chance of success for women undergoing IVF or other fertility procedures. The higher the AMH level, the more follicles in the ovary.[19, 20]

Zone 2

Early perimenopause and short/long menstrual cycles

In Zone 2, you are in your late 30s or older and are starting to experience a change in the regularity of your menstrual cycles. In fact, the hallmark of Zone 2 is *inconsistency*. Some women feel physically and emotionally inconsistent as well! The cycle inconsistency can be described as a marked change in the timing of menstrual periods, such that the interval between periods can vary from between 14 and 50 days. Some women experience having a period 'twice a month' and some say they 'never stop bleeding'. The inconsistency in the *timing* of menstrual periods has to do with a disturbance in the *timing of ovulation*. The blood hormone levels in my Ph.D. study showed that this disturbance is often due to the *overlapping* of ovulatory menstrual cycles, a phenomenon we called 'cycle stacking' or '**LOOP** (luteal out-of-phase) **cycles**'. It is when a new menstrual cycle starts during the luteal phase of the previous cycle. So, a new cycle starts before the previous has finished and this allows it to 'stack up' on top of the previous one. I found that these **LOOP cycles** were caused by more frequent ovulation episodes, and this was *the* breakthrough finding from my Ph.D. study.[21]

LOOP cycles have complex origins, but what is important for women to know is that they can occur in 30% or more of women during the perimenopause. When LOOP cycles occur, they can lead to higher-than-normal estrogen levels. Why? Because wherever the two cycles overlap, we know that at least two dominant follicles are developing in the ovaries at the same time. The estrogen produced by these dominant follicles can cause a two-fold or more increase in circulating levels of estrogen. These high estrogen levels, although transient, can lead to heavy menstrual bleeding, migraine headaches, weight gain, sleep disturbance, irritability, and sometimes abdominal bloating.

It is likely that LOOP cycles are caused by rising levels of FSH, but other age-related changes in the ovarian follicles may also be playing a role. Not all women experience LOOP cycles as a result of the rise in FSH, but most women are likely to have an increase in ovarian follicle (particularly dominant follicle) activity that can markedly increase estrogen levels. Some women only experience a lengthening of their menstrual cycles and as soon as they skip a cycle or their menstrual cycle interval reaches 60 days, they know they have reached Zone 3. Having longer menstrual cycles can be accompanied by either heavier or lighter than usual menstrual blood loss.

Sara: One of my Zone 2 patients

Sara came to see me and told me that she thought there must be something wrong with her uterus. An ultrasound imaging of her uterus hadn't shown any abnormalities, but she was still worried about cancer. She was only 46 and up until about six months before, she had been having regular periods. She told me that suddenly her periods came twice a month. She said some months, she would get two menstrual periods 10-14 days apart, and other months she would have just one as usual. She also reported that bleeding was at times very heavy and at other times quite light. She also had sore breasts and an expanding waistline and had begun having a few night-time waking episodes. She said she felt otherwise okay.

I explained to Sara that her menstrual bleeding woes were typical for women who were in the perimenopause. I told her that depending on how frequent and heavy her bleeding became, we could discuss further investigations. I also reassured her that having menstrual periods twice a month was highly unlikely to be from uterine cancer and instead was most likely due to LOOP cycles and more frequent ovulation. I estimated that she may experience these more frequent menstrual bleeds for six months or so, after which time they would resolve. In the meantime, she was interested to learn *why* she had such frequent bleeding and how she could help reduce it. I will cover the approach I took with Sara in **Section Three**.

Zone 3

Late perimenopause and long, infrequent menstrual cycles

In Zone 3, you will normally be in your late 40's or older and are starting to experience gaps of at least 60 days between menstrual periods. Once in Zone 3, women have around a 90% chance of experiencing their final menstrual period within the following 12 months. Even after entering Zone 3 however, some women can briefly resume regular menstrual cycles and even experience cycle-stacking and excessive menstrual bleeding. Two of the Zone 3 patients in my study had two periods in a month (with LOOP cycles) after having no period for two or three months. This is all part of the unpredictability of the perimenopause.

Typical menstrual cycle and hormone features in Zone 3 include:

- infrequent menstrual bleeding with variable blood loss
- infrequent ovulation and ovulatory cycles
- high FSH detected on routine blood hormone testing in *most* women
- either low or high estrogen levels detected on routine blood hormone testing in *some* women
- low progesterone levels when not having an ovulatory cycle.

It is worth noting that some women don't experience an obvious change in their menstrual cycles before their final menstrual period. In terms of the Zones, these women effectively move from Zone 1 to Zone 4 directly, without experiencing Zones 2 or 3. Also, if you are aged 40 or younger and are experiencing features consistent with Zone 3 or Zone 4, you could be experiencing premature menopause and should see your doctor to be tested and assessed for the need for hormone therapy.

I cover hormone therapies thoroughly in **Section Three**.

Bet: One of my Zone 3 patients

Bet was a 48-year-old patient who came to see me with irregular and heavy bleeding, headaches, sleep disturbance, anxiety, and irritability. About two months prior to seeing me, she didn't have a period for some 80 days. This put Bet into Zone 3. After her 80-day cycle, she experienced three menstrual periods in short succession over the following six weeks. By the time she saw me, she was having another period after a further break from bleeding of about 46 days. She told me that the three short cycles together were fairly heavy and accompanied by severe headaches and feeling very irritable. Prior to this, during her 80-day cycle, she had felt okay, but she was starting to feel some hot flushing. She said she seemed to be getting increasingly irritable no matter what her cycles were doing.

Bet is in Zone 3 and is experiencing typical symptoms of both high estrogen with more frequent ovulation/periods and low estrogen with less frequent ovulation/periods. Bet was keen to try menopausal hormone therapy (MHT) for her hot flushes, and I agreed this was a reasonable first-up strategy. MHT was bound to help ease Bet's hot flushing, but she was unlikely to get any relief from her episodic heavy bleeding. Given her long intermenstrual intervals between the frequent bleeds, it was likely she wasn't far off her final menstrual period. After explaining this and the reasons her periods were 'all over the place', she felt more at ease. She also felt more motivated to get into some of the dietary, lifestyle, and other strategies that I recommended. She was grateful for the information, because she had already been prescribed birth control pills for the heavy bleeding. She wasn't keen to take them because she hadn't tolerated them in the past and was worried about their side effects at her age. I will discuss more about the treatment strategies that I prescribed for Bet in **Section Three**.

More on LOOP cycles in Zone 2 and Zone 3

Because the finding of LOOP cycles originated from my Ph.D. study, I wanted to take the opportunity to illustrate how they fit into reproductive aging. In **Figure 5**, I have used stylized tracings of estrogen levels from a series of menstrual cycles from five individual women. The estrogen patterns for a young woman are shown at the TOP and below this, the patterns for women in Zones 1, 2, 3, and 4 respectively. Each series of cycles shown horizontally from left to right represents about five months. Feel free to look back at **Figure 1** to remind yourself of the pattern of estrogen levels throughout a normal menstrual cycle. *Only* the estrogen secretion patterns are shown as it would be an excessively busy figure if any other hormone patterns had been included.

Because LOOP cycles are a relatively new discovery and because no detailed hormone studies to date have been performed to duplicate the findings, few women's health or other doctors are informed about them. If women themselves know about them, they can be reassured that if their menstrual cycle patterns are 'all over the place', they are likely normal and don't need immediate investigation for other sinister causes. They can be reassured that they are caused by the expected disruption in ovulation and may cause frequent heavy bleeding for a limited time before menopause. They can also be reassured that they are a *normal* part of reproductive aging. Women can also help educate their doctors about them by giving them a copy of this book!

Figure 5: Estrogen secretion patterns in a series of menstrual cycles

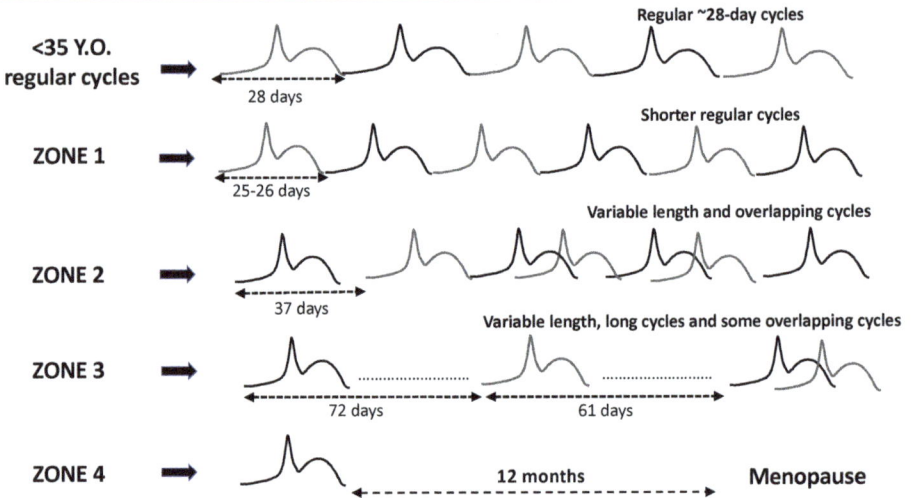

Figure Key:
TOP: <35-year-old woman with regular 28-day cycles
2nd row from TOP: Zone 1 woman with regular but slightly shorter 25-day cycles
3rd row: Zone 2 woman with a long 37-day cycle, then a normal length cycle, followed by two LOOP cycles, then a normal cycle
4th row: Zone 3 woman with a 72-day cycle, followed by 61-day cycle, followed by two LOOP cycles
5th row: Zone 4 woman showing her final menstrual period.

Zone 4

Menopause, no more menstrual cycles

In Zone 4, you have usually reached your late 40s or early 50s and you have not had a menstrual period for 12 months. This means you have most likely stopped ovulating, even though you still have a few-hundred ovarian follicles left in your ovaries that can continue to produce estrogen for a period of time.

Typical hormone features in Zone 4 include:

- no ovulation and no menstrual cycles
- variable but low estrogen and low progesterone levels
- high FSH and LH levels.

In Zone 4, although ovulation and menstrual cycling has stopped, the ovaries are still producing a small amount of estrogen from the remaining ovarian follicles. It varies, but after the final menstrual period, ovaries produce low-level estrogen for a year or so after menopause. This low level of estrogen production may help to reduce the low-estrogen symptoms that women experience at menopause. If you have just reached Zone 4, for example, and require surgery to remove your ovaries, you may well suffer from sudden and severe low estrogen symptoms after the surgery. This is because of the sudden loss of estrogen. Women who have recently reached menopause and are having their ovaries removed are often not warned of this because doctors forget or are not aware that, the menopausal ovary produces a low but variable level of estrogen for a year or so after the final menstrual period.

Tina: One of my Zone 4 patients

The final menstrual period was something one of my patients, Tina, had looked forward to for about four years. Tina had endured heavy periods on a semi-regular basis for at least four years before they finally stopped. She came to me some 16 months after her last menstrual period because she wanted my opinion on whether she should be taking hormone therapy. She was having hot flushes and was waking a lot at night but wasn't sure about taking estrogen since her estrogen levels had been so high a few years before. She had also heard that she would have to take a 'progestin' and was worried about the effect of these on her mood and her risk of breast cancer. She felt she was becoming increasingly anxious about not sleeping and the fact that she wasn't as sharp in her work as a financial market researcher. She had heard how important sleep was in the prevention of dementia. Her mother had died at age 72 from Alzheimer's disease.

If you are in Zone 4, then you are in the most talked-about Zone, the menopause. There seems to be endless discussions on when and how long to prescribe menopausal hormone therapy (MHT) and the research information has become increasingly complex. In addition, health professionals have differing opinions on how to interpret the growing body of research data and how to apply it to their individual patients. I enjoy the process of discussing MHT with patients, because the decision to treat is just as much about them as it is about the research data. Research data alone cannot give me all the answers I need to help patients make informed decisions. The initial discussion with Tina centered around her fears and anxiety, her lack of sleep, and the hot flushes. It was reassuring for Tina to learn she didn't have a positive family history of breast cancer and had no other risk factors such as obesity, diabetes, or heavy alcohol consumption. The next discussion was on the various forms of MHT and the fact that we could use a transdermal estrogen patch along with a human-equivalent progesterone hormone instead of a synthetic progestin. Her management plan is discussed further in **Section Three**.

Ovulation and progesterone

Ovulation can be confirmed by capturing a high progesterone blood level during the luteal phase of a menstrual cycle. If your menstrual cycles are *regular* and consistently between 26-29 days long however, you can presume that you are ovulating during most of your menstrual cycles and you don't need to have this confirmed unless for specific reasons. In my Ph.D. study, I measured blood hormone levels three times a week, and I found that *all* women in all age groups who had 26-29-day cycles were ovulating. Other studies have estimated that ovulation occurs in only 60-70% of normal length cycles.[22] In these studies, the progesterone was only measured on a single occasion during the luteal phase, so a peak level could have been missed.[22] In general, women are less likely to ovulate within the first 2-5 years of reproductive life and towards the end of their reproductive life after reaching Zone 3. You are also less likely to be ovulating when you don't have any menstrual periods. Reasons for absent menstrual periods include being severely underweight, medically ill or highly stressed, or when vigorously training for any type of excessive competitive sport such as an ultra-marathon, triathlon, or similar.

Knowing when ovulation is occurring is useful for women because in many ways it is a sign of health. Women who don't often ovulate may not develop as good a peak bone mass (and strength) as they could have if they were ovulating regularly.[23] This may have something to do with the fact that their bones don't get exposed to high cycling levels of both estrogen and progesterone. Progesterone, in addition to estrogen, promotes the formation and maintenance of optimal peak bone mass.[24] Reaching a high peak bone mass is important because the higher the peak bone mass in early life, the lower the chance of bone fractures later in life. Progesterone also helps prevent the abnormal build-up of the lining of the uterus (endometrium) and it also is important for maintaining optimal sleep and mood.[25]

Some women want to know whether they are producing sufficient levels of progesterone. This is usually only an issue if there are difficulties falling pregnant. Older midlife women, however, may want to know whether low progesterone may be causing symptoms. We will review some of these symptoms in the next section. In my Ph.D. study, progesterone was lower in women aged 45 or older than in women in their 20s.[12] My study, however, was a small one, and the large, detailed studies on blood progesterone levels needed to confirm my findings haven't been performed yet.

Pregnancy in midlife

Many women prefer, for many reasons, to delay starting a family until their late 30s. By this time, however, there may already be a significant reduction in their ability to get pregnant.[26] I illustrated this reduction in fertility at midlife at the 'down-turn' point in the number of ovarian follicles in **Figure 4**. Follicle *aging* appears to be a key factor in reduced fertility, via a disruption in the follicles' genetic material and its inbuilt 'anti-oxidant' capacity.[27] Nevertheless, there is always a chance of becoming pregnant when you are still ovulating, so unfortunately, contraception at midlife is still a requirement. I will discuss this further in **Section Three**.

If pregnancy in your late 30s and 40s is your aim, depending on the individual, there is still a reasonable chance of pregnancy if you are still in Zone 1. By Zone 2 or later however, you are well on the way to running out of ovarian follicles and fertility is diminishing fast. You can increase your chances of conception by knowing *when* the most 'productive' time to have intercourse is. Timing with your ovulation is crucial. While semen can last 5-7 days in the uterus and fallopian tubes after intercourse, an egg or ovum must 'meet her partner' within 24-30 hours of being expelled from the ovary. If she is kept waiting any longer, she simply passes out (literally) and is no longer available to couple with a sperm. So, your best option is to plan to have intercourse during the few days before and at the time of ovulation, a time when many women feel more 'receptive' anyway.

Even at midlife, many women can also increase the chance of getting pregnant through becoming healthier. If you are obese, you smoke, or live a stressful lifestyle, simple interventions like a nutritious diet, regular exercise, and relaxation techniques can improve fertility. Although there are no clinical studies to date to scientifically prove this, the scientific and anecdotal evidence of improved fertility through improving health is summarized comprehensively in *The Better Baby Book* by Dr. Lana and Dave Asprey.[28] I have witnessed women who have come to me with irritable bowel syndrome and infertility fall pregnant after we work through the dietary and other factors that promote optimal gut health. I will cover this in the dietary intervention parts of **Section Three**.

Testosterone levels at midlife

Testosterone is produced by the ovaries and the adrenal glands (the glands that sit on top of your kidneys). It is often only thought to be important in men, but it also plays an important role in women, including in musculoskeletal health, mood, skin, and sexuality. Women have 10 to 20-fold less testosterone at any given age and the levels tend to peak in their mid-20s, after which time, they gradually fall to low levels by menopause. There doesn't appear to be any significant fall in testosterone levels between Zone 1 and Zone 4 and levels are highly variable between women.[29] In fact, some recent research suggests that testosterone related hormones like DHEA may increase during perimenopause and may underlie the sudden sprouting of coarse facial hair that some women experience.[30] Before menopause, testosterone is produced by ovarian follicles and after menopause, it is mainly produced by the adrenal glands.[31]

I usually only request blood testosterone measurements in women who have recently reached menopause and who are complaining of symptoms that suggest it could be low. If a menopausal woman has symptoms of low testosterone and has very low blood levels, she may be a candidate for the careful addition of testosterone to the usual estrogen/progesterone hormone therapy. Women with polycystic ovary syndrome tend to have high testosterone and testosterone-related hormones, but this disorder usually becomes evident early in reproductive life. Occasionally, I have diagnosed it in a midlife woman, and this has been important because it is a condition that is linked to diabetes and is highly treatable with lifestyle interventions and a medication called metformin.[32]

Testing your hormones at midlife

Because the usual hormonal ups and downs are often exaggerated in midlife, it is worth knowing that while hormone testing can be useful in some circumstances, it is certainly not the 'be-all and end-all' in terms of answering midlife women's health questions. I use blood hormone testing as part of my initial assessment to exclude uncommon medical conditions and to perform a one-off check of the woman's reproductive hormones. I also sometimes measure blood levels of estrogen at the initiation of hormone therapy and luteal phase progesterone levels when checking for ovulation.

Can hormone testing determine whether your hormones are 'in balance'? Many women expect that hormone testing will tell them whether their hormones are *'balanced'* or not. Unfortunately, there are no standardized definitions or criteria that signify whether someone has *'balanced hormones'*, regardless of whether the testing is via blood, urine or saliva. The normal peaks and troughs in hormones throughout the menstrual cycle also make testing for 'balance' unreliable. I favor the term 'hormonal health' rather than hormonal 'balance' and in my experience, the best indicator of a woman's hormone health is if she feels fit, healthy, and happy. This is why I emphasize taking a detailed history of symptoms every time I see a patient, because it guides me as to where they are at in terms of their hormones. I will explain these symptoms at length in **Section Two**, and outline what each symptom may indicate with regard to hormone levels.

The two most common hormones that health professionals refer to as being in or out of 'balance' are estrogen and progesterone. One could say that a kind of 'hormonal balance' occurs between these two hormones within the lining of the uterus (endometrium), where estrogen acts to thicken the endometrium and progesterone acts to oppose it. It is more common to monitor the endometrial thickness with ultrasonography, rather than using hormone measurements. Whether or not an ideal 'balance' between estrogen and progesterone exists *elsewhere* in women's bodies, for example in the brain, blood vessels, and nervous system, remains unknown. Other hormones are also involved in the 'balance' between estrogen and progesterone, and they include testosterone, cortisol and the thyroid hormones. The relationship between all these hormones is highly complex, so trying to discern whether a patient is in or out of balance is somewhat difficult. It is a good thing the body knows what it is doing in this regard!

It is also worth bearing in mind that the more experienced a practitioner is, the less they will rely on hormone testing when working through your individual health issues and needs. Experienced practitioners adjust your hormone therapy according to changes in your symptoms, rather than by over-interpreting 'numbers' on multiple hormone tests. My advice is to avoid practitioners who offer extensive (and expensive) hormonal testing to tell you whether you are in or out of 'balance' and/or to adjust your hormone treatment, especially if you have concerns about the costs involved in the consultation.

The above reasons are why I avoid using terminology like 'balancing' or 're-balancing' or 'restoring' hormones when explaining my patients' health and hormone issues. Where I think the *concepts* of 'balance' and 'restoration' are useful in women's health, is when explaining the ways in which you can help your body 'balance' its own hormones and 'restore' itself to optimal health. Nevertheless, hormone therapies can be enormously helpful in alleviating the symptoms that many midlife and menopausal women experience as a result of changes in their hormones.

Can hormone testing determine whether you have 'estrogen dominance'?
Many women in my practice will have read something about 'estrogen dominance', a term that implies there is a disruption in the usual 'hormone balance', allowing estrogen to 'dominate' over progesterone or other hormones. The obvious situation is when there is no ovulation and therefore no rise in luteal phase progesterone. In effect, this causes estrogen to rise *relative to* progesterone. It may also occur in ovulatory menstrual cycles where estrogen is higher than usual, and progesterone is lower than usual (as described earlier in Zones 1 to 3). I don't use the term 'estrogen dominance' in my practice and instead explain to women where it is appropriate, that they may have *'estrogen excess'*. This situation is common in late reproductive age and perimenopause because of the increase in FSH stimulating the ovarian follicles (including the dominant follicle) to secrete more estrogen. In fact, I published a review article with Professor Claude Hughes about how this increase in estrogen during the menopause transition is likely a possible risk factor for the development of estrogen-dependent cancers.[33] Some

women in midlife and perimenopause can also get symptoms of lower than usual progesterone with or without symptoms of excess estrogen. In **Section Two**, I outline the symptoms associated with 'excess estrogen' and low progesterone, and in **Section Three** how to manage them using the *Estrogen Clearing* and *Progesterone Support* programs and hormone therapies.

The pitfalls of hormone testing and the 'normal range'

Both the time of day and the day of month greatly influence the outcome of any blood hormone level test result, especially if menstrual cycles are *irregular*. Blood hormone levels also vary widely from cycle to cycle in the same woman. Another issue is that hormone levels vary greatly *between* women, and although two women may have very different hormone levels, they both can be considered 'normal'. Some women are what I call 'low-estrogen' women, and others are 'high-estrogen' women. Regardless, their estrogen measurements will typically be within the normal range or 'expected range'. I have noticed however that some high-estrogen women who are experiencing high estrogen symptoms can show higher than normal levels, especially at midlife. More on high and low estrogen symptoms in **Section Two**.

It is worth knowing what 'normal' or 'expected' hormone levels are, so I will explain this. Blood hormone levels are always compared with expected values (the scientific term is *reference range*). For example, if hormone measurements are taken in the first half of the menstrual cycle (follicular phase), the expected estrogen level is somewhere between 230 and 1310 pmol/L (North American equivalent units would be 63-360 pg/mL). If the measurement was taken in the *second* half of the menstrual cycle (luteal phase), the expected estrogen level is somewhere between 180 and 840 pmol/L and the 'expected' progesterone level is between 15 and 63 nmol/L.

Right away, it is clear that 'balancing' hormones like estrogen and progesterone using blood measurements isn't going to be easy or accurate. The measurements can only really tell us that yes, enough estrogen is being produced, and yes, it appears progesterone is being produced (or not) and ovulation must have taken place (or not). On deeper inspection of the expected levels of estrogen and progesterone, the large difference in circulating levels between the two is obvious. See how a 'pmol' is used for estrogen levels and a 'nmol' is used for progesterone. This means that during the luteal phase, progesterone levels are normally some 100-500 times higher than estrogen. At other times, it may only be 10 times higher, and during menopause, it may even be lower than estrogen. And this is all 'normal'.

In practice, if I suspect that a woman may be entering menopause or they complain of menopause-type symptoms, I will measure both FSH and sometimes LH. You can refer back to **Table 1** (on **page 5**), to remind yourself of these two hormones produced in the pituitary. The FSH will usually not be elevated in Zone 1 or Zone 2, but when it is, it can be a sign that the last menstrual period is not far off. In Zone 3, the FSH is more likely to be elevated, but it can be high or low, especially if you measure it during highly *irregular* cycles. In Zone 4, the FSH is most likely to be elevated, and the higher the level, the closer the final menstrual period is likely to be. As mentioned earlier, testosterone measurements are usually only done after menopause, although sometimes they can be done in midlife women who complain of symptoms suggestive of low testosterone. Anti-Müllerian hormone (AMH) measurements are usually only taken in fertility assessments but can also be used to predict the final menstrual period. Inhibin B levels are mainly investigated in research and are rarely measured in the clinical setting.

NOTE: one nanomole (nmol) is 1,000,000,000th of a mole, and a picomole (pmol) is 1,000,000,000,000th of a mole, or 1000th of a nanomole.

Hormone measurements using urine tests

The other hormone test that I use in my practice is *dried urine hormone testing*.[34] These tests are very easy to perform and can be taken in the comfort of one's own home using mailable test-kits. The test-kits allow for urine hormone levels to be sampled across a single day or across an entire menstrual cycle, the latter being known as cycle mapping.

The single-day format of urine testing can be used in any Zone to give information about estrogen and progesterone production, hormone breakdown products, stress hormone levels, and other hormones such as melatonin. The third-daily urine measurements throughout a single menstrual cycle (called 'cycle mapping') is also useful for women with regular menstrual cycles who are looking for more accurate information on their cyclical estrogen and progesterone levels. I have found cycle mapping useful in Zone 1 and Zone 2 patients who are complaining of either high estrogen or low progesterone symptoms. I will discuss these symptoms in **Section Two**. Compared to the blood hormone measurements, urine hormone measurements are less dependent on the time/day of the sample being taken, because each level gives an estimate of the hormone production over the *previous* 6-24 hours (depending on how many samples are taken during a single day). One major drawback of the dried urine testing is the expense. In Australia, for example, the cost varies from between $300 and $600.

Another method of urine hormone testing that was established in the research community some years before the advent of dried urine testing, is using a 24-hour urine collection. This is a robust and standardized technique that is used in clinical research, but it is rarely used in clinical practice. It is the main method for measuring hormones in the ongoing North American population-based Study of Women Across the Nation or 'SWAN' study.[35]

Hormone testing using saliva

Another way to measure hormone levels is by taking samples of saliva. Compared to other methods however, salivary hormone levels are unreliable, and estrogen and progesterone levels have not been shown to correlate well with blood levels. Salivary *cortisol* levels, however, do correlate well with blood levels and this is often the preferred method to measure cortisol amongst clinicians who measure this hormone on a regular basis. Cortisol is the body's most important stress hormone and I use the salivary cortisol testing when my patients have persistent and unexplained fatigue. The saliva is measured at 4-5 specified times during a single day to demonstrate both the levels and the pattern of secretion across the day and night.

Hormone testing in Zone 1

Although there are no 'diagnostic' hormone tests for women in Zone 1, it is not unreasonable to run a series of initial blood hormone tests along with other appropriate tests if there are worrisome symptoms. Even if there are symptoms suggestive of high estrogen (see **Section Two**), it is unusual to find abnormalities in the blood hormone levels because, as I have mentioned previously, any changes in estrogen and progesterone in Zone 1 tend to be subtle. Nevertheless, if you visit your healthcare provider for any reason, it is entirely reasonable for them to arrange blood hormone measurements as a one-off check-up for abnormalities. Hormones requested may include FSH, LH, estrogen, progesterone, testosterone, sex-hormone binding globulin, prolactin, and anti-Müllerian hormone. For all these hormones, except progesterone, the blood measurement is usually taken on cycle-day 2-5 of a menstrual cycle. If an assessment of ovulation is needed, a progesterone measurement is usually taken between cycle-day 19 and 21 day of a menstrual cycle (during the mid-luteal phase).

A hormone measurement taken on cycle-day 2-5 of the menstrual cycle may turn up a mildly elevated FSH, the first sign of reproductive aging and that progression through the perimenopause is not far off. If I suspect high estrogen symptoms in a Zone 1 woman, I might request a cycle-day 2-5 and a cycle-day 19-21 estrogen measurement, especially if she was interested in further discussions about health programs, like the Estrogen Clearing Program (see **Section Three**). If I suspect low progesterone symptoms in a patient, I may also suggest she do cycle-mapping testing using the dried urine testing. This would be more revealing in terms of the hormonal dynamics throughout her entire menstrual cycle and perhaps increase the chances of differentiating her test results from the 'expected or normal'.

Hormone testing in Zone 2 and Zone 3

Making sense of hormone testing is particularly challenging once your menstrual cycles become irregular and/or more frequent in Zone 2 and Zone 3. As I explained in **Section One**, estrogen can rise to higher and more frequent peaks in Zone 2 and higher but less frequent peaks in Zone 3. This reflects the more frequent ovulation during LOOP cycles that can occur in Zone 2 and the less frequent ovulation in Zone 3. On the other hand, estrogen can at times drop to *less than normal levels*, especially in Zone 3. This may lead to symptoms of both high estrogen and low estrogen, some of which can occur at the same time within a single menstrual cycle (I explain this further in **Section Two**).

The unpredictable nature of the high peaks of estrogen and ovulation can mean that blood measurements taken during Zone 2 and Zone 3 are unreliable in determining whether your FSH, estrogen or progesterone are lower or higher than 'normal'. Generally speaking, if a measurement is taken on cycle-day 2-5, FSH is likely to be elevated and if a measurement is taken on cycle-day 19-21, estrogen may be elevated, especially in Zone 2 during a LOOP cycle. Once you start getting frequent menstrual bleeding in Zone 3, it becomes increasingly challenging to time blood hormone measurements to achieve meaningful results.

Hormone testing in Zone 4

In Zone 4, blood hormone measurements usually reveal an elevated FSH, a low estrogen and a very low progesterone. The reliability of capturing a high FSH in Zone 4 women means it can be used to 'diagnose' menopause in women who don't have a uterus and who therefore will not experience a 'final menstrual period'. If you are 45 years or older, don't have a uterus, and you have a blood FSH level of 25 IU/L or greater, it means you have likely reached menopause or Zone 4. If you are less than 45 years old, this test should be repeated at another time to confirm an elevated FSH, and thus menopause.

Blood measurements of estrogen are not used to determine whether you are close to or at menopause, as estrogen can remain high and variable for some time after menopause. If a Zone 4 woman in my practice is keen to find out more about her hormones and wants more input about her health, I offer the dried urine testing, because it is easy to do, and gives information about the level of hormone production, her ability to clear her own hormones, the ability to clear additional hormones (if taking hormone therapy), the level and pattern of stress hormones, and the production of testosterone and related hormones. I discuss more about why I use this test in **Section Three**, when I discuss what to do about your hormone measurement results.

What about other hormone tests?

In my practice, I always check for thyroid problems, particularly if a woman is complaining of unexplained fatigue, excess weight gain, hair loss, aches and pains, or heart palpitations. The hormonal changes that occur between Zone 1 and Zone 4 are a recognized trigger for autoimmune disease, and autoimmune disease of the thyroid can affect up to one in 15-20 women by midlife.[36] It is called *Hashimoto's thyroiditis* or *lymphocytic thyroiditis*. Even if the initial thyroid test, which measures thyroid-stimulating-hormone (TSH), is normal, I check whether any thyroid antibodies are present. These antibodies are called anti-peroxidase and anti-thyroglobulin antibodies, and they can sometimes greatly reduce the optimal functioning of the thyroid gland. Many women in my practice with Hashimoto's disease can reduce the adverse effects of it through the management of chronic gut symptoms, food intolerance, and mycotoxin illness (mold-related illness).

Hashimoto's thyroiditis is linked to high blood pressure and low vitamin D, which makes sense because both conditions are associated with excess *inflammation*. Excess body inflammation can lead to high blood pressure by causing abnormalities within the inside of blood vessels (called endothelial dysfunction) that, over time, can lead to cardiovascular disease.[37, 38] Having a low vitamin D can have a number of adverse effects on the body. Among them is a dysregulation in the recognition of 'self' and 'non-self', leading to an increased susceptibility to autoimmune diseases.[39] For this reason, I measure vitamin D in all women who have thyroid abnormalities and make sure they get targeted sunshine therapy and/or supplementation to keep their Vitamin D in the upper normal range. Low Vitamin D is one of the easiest barriers to full health that can be easily overcome.

What can you do *without* hormone testing

If you are not in a position to get blood or dried urine hormone measurements done, you can still get a good idea about the hormonal changes occurring in your body. The key to this is being able to 'read' what I call *the language of your body*, and this is what you can begin to do after reading **Section Two**. In this section, I aim to give you a newfound understanding about how your symptoms are linked to changes in your hormones. It turns out that you may even be able to 'read' your body better than blood hormone testing, because as I have explained, blood tests only capture a brief 'hormone moment in time' and can miss the hormonal rollercoaster that is really taking place. Your hormones could be reaching much higher and falling much lower than normal for you, even while your single blood hormone measurement indicates everything is perfectly 'normal'. So, I invite you to read on.

Your Zone:

Your hormones and symptoms explained

In this section, you can use the information from **Section One** to explore the hormonal changes that could explain some of your midlife symptoms. If your symptoms don't include hot flushes or night sweats, chances are this book will provide the only explanation you can find. In fact, midlife symptoms other than hot flushes are barely studied, let alone understood. I was not aware of any non-menopausal symptoms unique to midlife women until I did my Ph.D. study. Not only did I then become aware of the symptoms, but I also realized the lack of explanation for them.

Here is what one woman said about midlife:

> In my early 40s I experienced the onset of disrupted sleep and a new edginess. I had a hard time feeling calm. At first, it didn't occur to me that my symptoms might be related to perimenopause because I was only 42 and still getting a monthly period. I associated perimenopause with hot flashes and skipped periods. I consulted the scientific research and learned about the late reproductive stage when periods are still coming monthly but starting to change subtly: shortening cycles, changes to amount of menstrual flow or number of days of flow. Although I didn't find much research on this stage, I did find Dr. Hale's work and two other research studies that supported the idea that changes begin for some people before menstrual irregularity.

The author of this paragraph in fact went on to publish a unique survey of midlife women and their symptoms.[18] Their results showed that although most midlife women with regular menstrual cycles expect to get symptoms with menopause, less than 15% of them expect to get them *before* menopause. **Figure 6** shows the results from Zone 1 women aged 35-56 (most women still had regular menstrual periods). The survey also found the symptoms seen in this figure were as common or more common in women in Zone 2, 3, or 4. Breast tenderness was more common in the Zone 1 women, but low mood, low libido, forgetfulness, and hot flushes were more common in the Zone 2, 3, or 4 women.

I investigated a number of other symptoms in my Ph.D. study, including itchiness, crawling sensations under the skin, joint pain, fatigue, bloating, headaches, and excessive menstrual blood loss, all of which were reported in Zone 1, 2, and 3 women. My aim was to determine if there was any association between symptoms and hormone changes. Unfortunately, the symptoms were too scattered across my small group of 77 women and the hormonal levels too variable for the data to reveal any significant links between symptoms and hormonal changes. What my Ph.D. study *did* tell me was just how challenging it is to research symptoms and hormonal changes in midlife women. This is perhaps the main reason why research on women's symptoms has been largely limited to Zone 4 women. In menopause, women no longer have the 'complex' hormonal ups and downs for researchers to account for.

Figure 6: Symptoms reported in women aged 35-56 with regular menstrual cycles

945-woman survey: Age 35-56 with 3-4 menstrual periods in the past 3 months

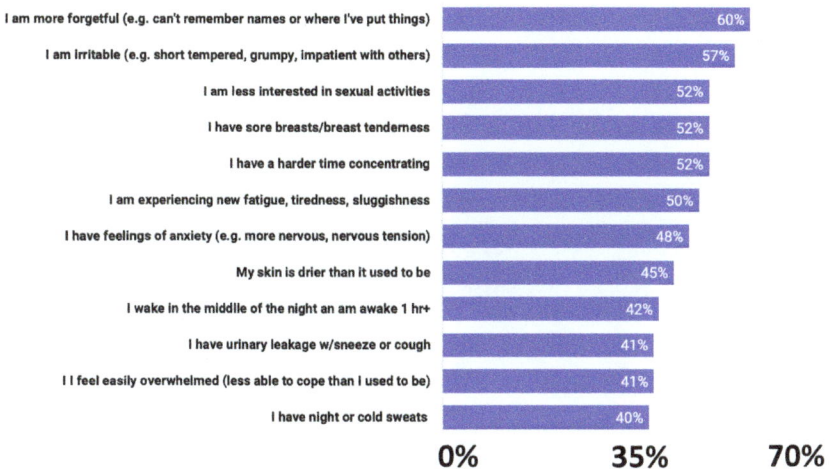

Symptom	Percentage
I am more forgetful (e.g. can't remember names or where I've put things)	60%
I am irritable (e.g. short tempered, grumpy, impatient with others)	57%
I am less interested in sexual activities	52%
I have sore breasts/breast tenderness	52%
I have a harder time concentrating	52%
I am experiencing new fatigue, tiredness, sluggishness	50%
I have feelings of anxiety (e.g. more nervous, nervous tension)	48%
My skin is drier than it used to be	45%
I wake in the middle of the night an am awake 1 hr+	42%
I have urinary leakage w/sneeze or cough	41%
I I feel easily overwhelmed (less able to cope than I used to be)	41%
I have night or cold sweats	40%

0%   35%   70%

Because of the paucity of clinical research studies in this area of women's health, many of my explanations in this book are derived from a combination of my clinical experience, my Ph.D. research and what I have learnt from the principles of functional medicine. They are also a result of gathering knowledge from listening to my patients closely and monitoring their responses to various diet, lifestyle, medications, and supplement interventions.

Jess: One of my Zone 1 patients

Remember Jess, the Zone 1 woman I mentioned in **Section One**? When Jess came to me for advice, she was 42 years old and had recent onset sleep disturbance, increased irritability, low mood, sore breasts, midriff weight gain, and heavy menstrual bleeding. In my clinical practice, these complaints are common in Zone 1 women. As you may recall, Zone 1 is when your follicle numbers start to fall *precipitously*. As I explained, this leads to a rise in FSH and estrogen and may also result in a fall in luteal-phase progesterone. These hormonal changes are subtle, and although clinical research to date has been unable to confirm whether they are linked to midlife symptoms, my clinical experience tells me they are likely to play a role. To be clear, many of Jess's symptoms may be influenced by factors other than changes in her hormones. For example, there may be several reasons for her irritability such as work stress, poor sleep, unrealized goals, or problems with her children's schoolwork, etc. So, it is worth remembering that your everyday life in addition to your hormones can influence how your body functions.

I am very much in favor of educating women about *how* your hormones can influence your symptoms and general health. Accordingly, this section is about recognizing how the changes in your hormones *can* change your body and influence your mood and mental health. I will cover each of the midlife symptoms listed below in **Table 2**. For each symptom, I have indicated how common it is in each Zone.

NOTE: if you don't have a uterus, have always had irregular periods or don't have menstrual periods for other reasons, your Reproductive Zone may become clear simply by noting the symptoms that you are experiencing and what underlying hormonal changes are likely to be occurring.

Table 2: Midlife symptoms according to your Zone

SYMPTOM	Zone 1 score	Zone 2 score	Zone 3 score	Zone 4 score
Heavy bleeding with regular periods	♦♦	♦♦♦	♦♦♦	—
Erratic, frequent periods	—	♦♦♦	♦♦	—
Uterine fibroids	♦♦	♦♦♦	♦♦♦	♦♦
Endometriosis	♦	♦	♦	—
Sleep disturbance	♦♦	♦♦	♦♦♦	♦♦♦
Abdominal bloating/discomfort and midriff weight gain	♦♦♦	♦♦♦	♦♦	♦
Breast swelling and swelling of extremities	♦♦♦	♦♦♦	♦♦	♦
Mastalgia, breast soreness	♦♦♦	♦♦♦	♦♦	♦
Headache and migraine (high estrogen)	♦♦♦	♦♦♦	♦	—
Headache and migraine (low estrogen)	—	—	♦♦	♦♦♦
Aches and pains	♦♦	♦♦♦	♦♦	♦♦♦
Irritability and anxiety	♦♦	♦♦♦	♦♦♦	♦♦♦
Low mood and depression	♦	♦♦	♦♦♦	♦♦♦
Premenstrual syndrome (PMS)	♦♦	♦♦♦	♦♦♦	—
Low libido	♦♦	♦♦	♦♦	♦♦
Forgetfulness and poor concentration	♦♦	♦♦	♦♦	♦♦
Hot flushes and night sweats	♦	♦	♦♦	♦♦♦
Vaginal dryness and vaginal pain	—	—	♦	♦♦♦
Recurrent urinary tract and vaginal infections	—	—	♦	♦♦♦
Painful bladder syndrome	♦	♦	♦	♦
Bone loss and osteoporosis	—	♦	♦♦	♦♦♦

KEY: '—' tends not to occur in this Zone; '♦' uncommon but can happen in this Zone; '♦♦' common in this Zone; '♦♦♦' very common in this Zone

Heavy bleeding with regular periods

Zone 1	Zone 2	Zone 3	Zone 4
♦♦	♦♦♦	♦♦♦	—

Heavy menstrual bleeding isn't talked about a lot by medical or non-medical people, so many women who have had heavy periods since menses think it is 'normal' until they have discussions with friends who have light periods. At least

20% of women will experience what they report as heavy menstrual periods or heavy menstrual 'flow'.[40] Whatever your 'normal' menstrual blood flow is, you, like many women, may experience an increase in menstrual flow at midlife. In fact, almost one in every three women experience increased menstrual blood flow after age 35 and/or during the transition to menopause.[41]

Blood loss during a menstrual period
In my Ph.D. study, I used *quantitative* blood loss calculations to explore the amount of blood lost during each of the women's menstrual periods. The amount of blood varied from around 2 mL to more than 250 mL (8.5 fl.oz). That's *a lot* of menstrual bleeding! Very few other studies have *quantitatively* measured blood loss, and instead have relied on women's descriptions of soaked pads and tampons or similar. One of the few other quantitative studies performed found that blood loss didn't exceed 120 mL in young women (with no structural abnormalities or bleeding diseases). In women older than 44-years-old, however, blood loss was observed to be a lot more variable and sometimes exceeded 230 mL.[42] It is worth noting that only about *one third* of the fluid that is passed through the vagina during a menstrual period is *pure* blood. About two thirds is comprised of non-blood bodily fluids. This proportion does however vary widely between women.

Your periods are 'heavy' by definition if you:
- bleed for more than 8 days in a menstrual period, OR
- pass visible clots of blood larger than 1.5 cm in diameter, OR
- need to change sanitary pads or tampons every hour, OR
- have to get up during the night to change pads or tampons, OR
- suddenly bleed through sanitary pads and clothing (flooding), OR
- have blood loss sufficient to reduce your quality of life.

If you don't fit into these criteria above, but feel your menstrual flow is heavy or has increased, it is still worth reading on to find out what hormonal and other factors are at play.

If you have *always* had excessive bleeding, it is advisable to get checked for a bleeding disorder like Von Willebrand's disease. Sometimes heavy menstrual bleeding is the only indication you may have of a bleeding disorder.

Menstrual bleeding comes from the inner lining of the uterus

The inner lining of the uterus is called the endometrium, and a close-up of the endometrium is shown in **Figure 7**. It shows from left to right, the changes that occur over a single menstrual cycle. The first half of the cycle is called the *follicular phase*, the second half is called the *luteal phase*. At the top, you can read the words for the different layers of the endometrium. You can see that the endometrium is at its thinnest just after the start of the menstrual period (5-8 mm thick) and is thickest in the middle of the luteal phase (12-15 mm thick). The endometrium initially builds up in thickness in response to rising estrogen, then in the second half of the cycle (luteal phase), the rising progesterone transforms it in readiness to receive a pregnancy. If a pregnancy doesn't occur, progesterone levels fall, and this fall triggers the breakdown of the endometrium leading to a menstrual period. This also signals the end of one menstrual cycle and the beginning of the next.

Figure 7: The uterine lining sheds during a menstrual period

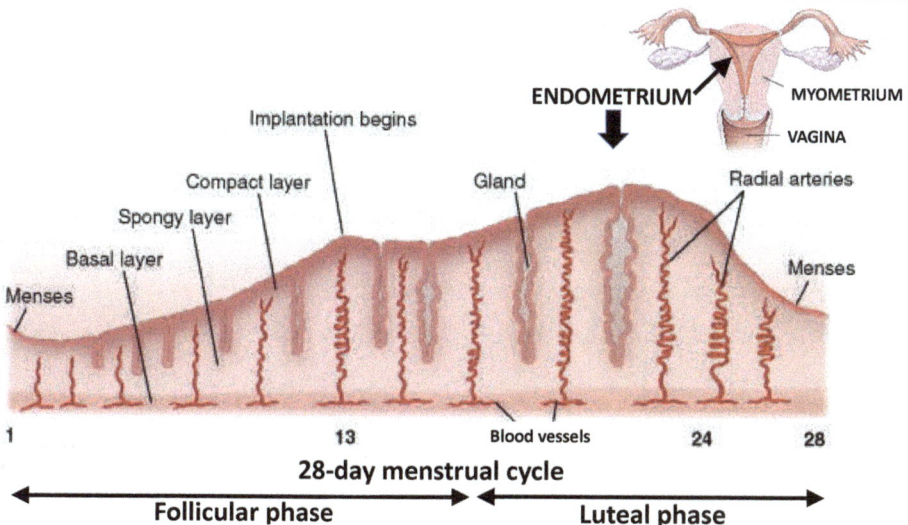

28-day menstrual cycle

Follicular phase   Luteal phase

During a menstrual period, the blood vessels and glands within the outer layers of the endometrium are discarded and those within the inner layer are retained to form the basis of the next menstrual cycle and another process of endometrial build up. Menstrual bleeding is a surprisingly complex process that is regulated by many factors within the endometrium itself and within the wider circulation. Many of these factors involve the promotion and the inhibition of *inflammation*.[43] The actions of progesterone tend to inhibit or counteract inflammation and when progesterone falls at the end of a menstrual cycle, it triggers a specific inflammatory process that leads to the shedding of the endometrium and blood loss.[44] In fact, this is why medications that inhibit inflammation can significantly reduce the amount of menstrual blood loss.[45] This also helps explain why dietary modifications that reduce whole-body inflammation can also reduce menstrual blood loss. I'll explain more about these in **Section Three**.

What determines how much you bleed?

There are factors other than inflammation that can cause heavy bleeding either in young adult life or midlife. One of the more obvious factors is higher than normal estrogen. My clinical observations have led me to believe that some women tend to produce more estrogen than expected or what is in the 'normal range', and I term them 'high-estrogen' women. High estrogen levels have been linked to heavy menstrual bleeding in a number of studies[46] including my own Ph.D. study where I found heavy menstrual bleeding occurred following some of the menstrual cycles where there was high estrogen with the 'LOOP cycles'.[47] I observed LOOP cycles in four of my Zone 2 women and seven of my Zone 3 women (**see page 16**). The excessive menstrual blood loss (greater than 200 mL) however, only occurred in the Zone 3 women. Remember, Zone 3 is when you start *skipping* menstrual periods.

You might ask *why* after reaching Zone 3, would some women bleed excessively. It is likely because of a combination of high estrogen levels and low progesterone levels. Remember skipped periods indicate that you haven't ovulated and if you haven't ovulated, you don't get the rise in progesterone. Without progesterone, the endometrium cannot undergo the normal buildup across the follicular and luteal phases. Also, without progesterone, estrogen causes the endometrium to become disordered, and if the endometrium is then exposed to a normal ovulatory cycle, the ensuing menstrual period can be extra-heavy and disruptive. In fact, changes in ovulation at midlife are likely to be the most common cause of heavy menstrual bleeding at midlife with structural problems such as non-cancerous polyps, benign tumors, fibroids and endometrial hyperplasia accounting for only 25-30% (covered later in this section).[48]Bleeding disorders such as Von Willebrand's disease likely account for less than 5% of heavy menstrual bleeding.[49]

Because most heavy bleeding in midlife women isn't due to a structural problem or a bleeding disorder, most women can benefit from intermittent hormonal or other medication in addition to select diet and lifestyle interventions. I have found the diet and lifestyle interventions can help greatly reduce blood loss, improve general wellbeing, and reduce the need for medication. These interventions are covered in **Section Three** when I introduce the Basic and Estrogen Clearing Programs.

Erratic, frequent periods

Zone 1	Zone 2	Zone 3	Zone 4
—	♦♦♦	♦♦	—

More frequent menstrual periods may mean your period comes every 25-26 days instead of 28-29 days (Zone 1), or it may mean you are getting them even more frequently, like every 14-20 days, almost twice a month. If you have a period twice a month, it's an indication that you may be experiencing LOOP cycles, which I covered at length in **Section One**. Both this and a slightly shortened cycle length in Zone 1 result from the hormonal changes that occur secondary to the accelerated loss of ovarian follicles. When menstrual cycles are normal for one month, then occur twice a month for 1-2 months before becoming 'normal' again, this is very typical of Zone 2.

It is worth mentioning here that no two women are the same in terms of how their menstrual cycles change between being normal length and stopping altogether at menopause. Some women don't notice any change at all until they realize that they haven't had a period for 3-4 months (and are not pregnant). These women have skipped Zones 2 and Zone 3 and have progressed directly from Zone 1 to Zone 4. In my experience, it is the 'high estrogen' women who tend experience Zone 2 and Zone 3 with erratic menstrual cycles and menstrual bleeding prior to moving on to Zone 4. If this is you, you should stay in touch with your healthcare provider on a regular basis in case they feel you need some medical screening tests including checks for blood-loss anemia. I cover some of the useful medical/surgical treatments in **Section Three**, as well as some of the helpful diet and lifestyle tips that I have found help to support patients through this time.

Sara: The Zone 2 patient mentioned in Section One

Remember Sara came to see me because she was concerned there may be something wrong with her uterus. She had suddenly started having a menstrual period twice a month, and they were becoming heavier and more painful. She was also waking up multiple times through the night feeling hot, and worrying about what was going on.

During the first consultation, I also found out that Sara had been a one-pack-a-day smoker until five years previously and that her mother had gone through menopause at age 45 (about six years earlier than the average). These two factors increased the likelihood that she herself would go through menopause some time in her mid-40s. Given Sara's menstrual cycle history and her slightly elevated FSH on blood testing, I explained to her that she was in Zone 2, the early perimenopause. I also gave her a brief explanation about why her periods were so erratic and it indeed signalled that menopause wasn't far off.

Sara went on to mention that she was also having some hot flushing and night sweats. This could indicate that her estrogen levels were, at times, very low, that her ovarian follicles were running low and that her final menstrual period was imminent. I gave her advice on how to track her menstrual periods so that at a review appointment, I could give her even more of an idea about how long she'd have to endure the more frequent menstrual bleeding.

When I saw Sara four months later, she showed me her menstrual cycle diary, which indicated that she had skipped a period the previous month. I checked with her about any other possible causes for this, such as excessive physical training, or a traumatic event such as the loss of a loved one, neither of which applied to her. I was then able to advise her that she had reached Zone 3, the final step before menopause. While she wasn't ecstatic about being menopausal, she was happy that her periods were lighter and less frequent. She also said that she had been experiencing more daytime hot flushes and was keen to talk about possible treatment for those. More on how we managed Sara's symptoms in **Section Three**.

Uterine fibroids

Zone 1	Zone 2	Zone 3	Zone 4
♦♦	♦♦♦	♦♦♦	♦♦

Fibroids, also called leiomyomas, are non-cancerous growths within the wall of the uterus that affect 70-80% of all women and can cause heavy and painful menstrual bleeding, especially in midlife.[50] While we don't know what causes them, they flourish and grow under the influence of estrogen.[51] They are very 'fibrous' in structure, hence their name. Up to 70% of Caucasian women and 80% of women of African descent have them in their uterus,[52] but only about one in three women will experience troublesome symptoms from them, and this is usually at midlife under the influence of rising estrogen levels.[53]

Common symptoms from fibroids:
- excessive bleeding and blood-loss anemia
- pelvic and back pain
- urinary frequency
- constipation and abdominal bloating
- infertility.

Factors that increase your risk of having problematic fibroids:

- African descent
- midriff obesity (central obesity)
- sedentary
- low vitamin D level (much more common in dark-skinned women)
- excess alcohol consumption
- exposure to excessive environmental estrogen-like chemicals or 'endocrine disrupters'.

If you are going to have a problem with fibroids at all, you will most likely have the problem after reaching Zone 1 or Zone 2, although fibroids can become symptomatic during any of the Zones. If you have troublesome fibroids, it may take 12 months or so *after* Zone 4 for severe symptoms to resolve. Thus, for those women who start having severe symptoms as early as Zone 1 or Zone 2, surgical removal may be the treatment of choice.[54]

Figure 8 shows a stylized figure of uterine fibroids. Fibroids are usually a rough spherical shape sitting either on the inside wall of the endometrium, within the muscle wall of the uterus or within the outer wall of the uterus. Sometimes fibroids can literally hang outside the wall of the uterus (*pedunculated* forms). Fibroids are easily seen on routine ultrasound examinations

Figure 8: Uterine fibroids (leiomyomas)

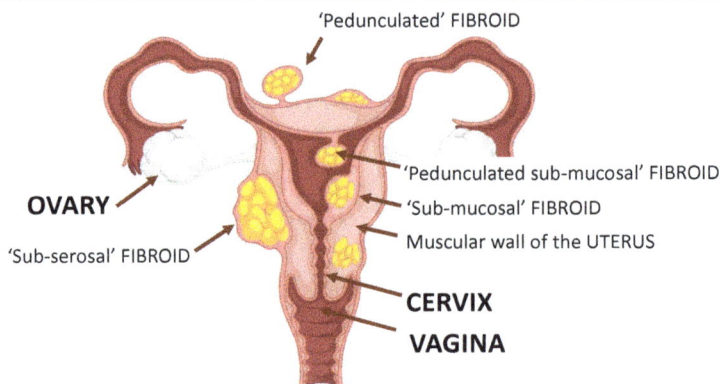

'Pedunculated' FIBROID

OVARY

'Sub-serosal' FIBROID

'Pedunculated sub-mucosal' FIBROID

'Sub-mucosal' FIBROID

Muscular wall of the UTERUS

CERVIX

VAGINA

of the pelvis. An ultrasound examination is an economical and easy imaging technique, that can be improved by using a trans-vaginal probe to image the uterus and endometrium instead of the normal ultrasound probe on the outside of the lower abdomen.

Endometriosis

Zone 1	Zone 2	Zone 3	Zone 4
◆	◆	◆	—

You have most likely heard about endometriosis, and you may have even suffered from it yourself. The severe debilitating menstrual cramping and pain typical of endometriosis affects 10-15% of women and although it doesn't preferentially affect midlife women, like fibroids, if you suffer from it at all, it doesn't tend to abate until *after* Zone 4. While hormones per se don't seem to *trigger* endometriosis, they do play a role in maintaining it, once it has formed. [55] While it remains unclear, the most important triggers for the formation endometriosis appear to be excess inflammation and a disruption in the normal function of the autonomic nervous system.[56, 57] Further clues about what can trigger its formation lie in the fact that it is linked to having other disorders like irritable bowel syndrome, autoimmune disease and some cancers such as ovarian and thyroid cancer.[58]

What is endometriosis exactly?

When you have endometriosis, your own endometrial lining has somehow formed smaller pieces of itself that have migrated outside of the uterus to other areas like the ovary, the pelvic cavity, the bowel, and the abdominal cavity. Having moved to these places, these pieces of endometrium build up and shed the same way the normal endometrium does inside the uterus. So, strangely enough, if you have endometriosis, you are menstruating all over the inside of your body! That doesn't sound great, and this is likely why women with endometriosis suffer from severe, sometimes debilitating menstrual pain, chronic pelvic and abdominal pain, pain on intercourse, pain on passing urine, and even infertility. All these symptoms are likely due to excess inflammation and the build-up of menstrual blood inside the body cavity with nowhere to go. Moreover, the combination of chronic pain and inflammation cause some women to be chronically unwell.

Given the role of inflammation in the formation of endometriosis and endometriosis-related pain, it makes sense that an important aspect of managing the disorder is to reduce inflammation. I always advise endometriosis patients to combine the anti-inflammatory and Estrogen Clearing eating programs with stress-reduction techniques. This combination is key to success in managing endometriosis, and often allows women to reduce their dependence on surgical interventions and medications.

My own experience with endometriosis:

There is a reason I offer women a diet and stress-reduction approach to endometriosis, and it's because of my own experience of having endometriosis in my early twenties. At the time, I was using a handful of pain and anti-inflammatory pills every time I had a period. The pain was severe for about twelve hours before the first day and didn't let up much until the end of cycle-day 3. The pain would cause me to vomit, and on a couple of occasions, I passed out. To my horror, on one occasion, I ended up in the emergency room in the hospital where I was working, which was not fun. I went through the usual tests to exclude anything serious, and all was okay. Thereafter, I started to educate myself more about endometriosis, what could be the causes, and what I could do about it myself. It seemed to me to be a multi-system disorder, but in the literature, it was often linked to a psychological problem. While we didn't have a lot of answers or solutions at the time, I was very wary of getting a 'psychological' label and, because there were only surgical options at the time, I avoided further investigations and didn't seek further medical advice.

I began reading more widely than just medical books and I came across one book called *A Women's Best Medicine*.[59] This book outlined reasonably straightforward steps to help manage the pain of endometriosis. As suggested,

I stepped up my meditation, took more warm baths, ate warm, cooked, well-seasoned meals, and enjoyed some regular relaxing warm-oil massages. All these steps were to supposedly help calm my nervous system which the authors referred to as 'reducing excess vata' (an Ayurvedic medicine approach). It was quite weird, because within a few months, I noticed the menstrual pain became much less severe, I stopped vomiting and never passed out again with pain. Beyond a year or so of maintaining most of the program, to my delight, I never again experienced anything but mild and brief period pain.

The Ayurvedic approach that had me calming my 'excess vata' relates to calming so-called chaotic 'nervous energy' inside the body. The Ayurvedic 'theory' about endometriosis in *A Women's Best Medicine* proposes that chaotic 'nervous energies' within the body can somehow 'pick up' the endometrium, causing it to move out of the uterus and into other areas within the pelvis and abdominal cavity. We know that endometrial tissue is highly hormone-responsive, but we don't know about it being 'energy-sensitive'. Even at that time, this theory or concept didn't seem too outlandish. After all, I felt a whole lot better and knew the diet/lifestyle changes I had made were bound to make a positive impact on my current and future health. I did realize that it would probably take many years for modern science to do justice to such theories with good quality studies, but that didn't stop me taking part in my successful one-person trial.

Many women who live a fast and stressful life probably resonate with the term 'chaotic energies'. We all know how much better we feel when we escape city chaos and set ourselves down in a comfortable, quiet place to simply 'sink into ourselves' while surrounded by nature and beauty. We are discovering more and more today about the science of the health benefits that can be gained from improving gut health, reducing stress, and emphasizing happiness and gratitude in our lives.[60, 61] These are all important aspects that women with endometriosis can address so they can look forward to more comfortable and better lives.

Sleep disturbance

Zone 1	Zone 2	Zone 3	Zone 4
♦♦	♦♦	♦♦♦	♦♦♦

You may have noticed that you don't *stay* asleep at night anymore, or you seem to wake up several times through the night either briefly or for longer periods. If this is you, you may have *'disturbed'* sleep.[62] Disturbed sleep affects up to 50% of women after age 40 and in an astonishing *half* of these women, the problem is severe and classified as *insomnia*.[63] Sleep and health studies clearly link poor sleep to poor health outcomes, so addressing your sleep is certainly a *priority* if you want to optimize your health in the future.[64] I had difficulties myself with disturbed sleep, and at times, still do. I, like most midlife women, had at least three factors contributing to my sleep problem, one of which was getting anxious about not sleeping! Even now, I continue to observe a number of 'sleep hygiene' practices to maintain sleep quality and quantity and I regularly monitor my progress using a sleep-tracker.

According to the large SWAN study in the US, episodes of night-time waking increase as we advance from Zone 1 to Zone 4, and it seems that sleep disturbance is worst around Zone 3 and Zone 4.[65, 66] This has been confirmed in some of the detailed polysomnogram sleep-laboratory studies, but not others.[67] These detailed studies that require laboratory conditions are necessarily small, so it may take many of these types of studies to clarify the relationship between reproductive Zone and sleep quality. Nevertheless, it seems that if you have sleep issues in Zone 1 and Zone 2, the issues are *three to four* times more likely to worsen in Zone 3 and Zone 4, especially if you are also experiencing hot flushes.[68]

Poor sleep at midlife has been found to be linked to having severe hot flushes and night sweats, a low libido, and low mood.[69] If you have been treated for depression before reaching Zone 1, you are also more likely to have sleep problems once you reach Zone 2 and beyond.[70] Not all studies, however, have been able to find a link between depression and sleep disturbance and unexpectedly, the link between anxiety and sleep is even less clear.[71]

If you have night-time hot flushing, you may have noticed that you don't wake up *because of a flush*, but you wake up *before* you flush. So, while the flush itself may not be waking you up, it is likely that the body and brain changes leading up to the flush *are*. These detailed studies also show that night-time flushing doesn't seem to occur during the rapid-eye-movement phase of sleep, or REM sleep. It is thought that this has to do with the partial shut-down of the heat regulation centered in the hypothalamus during REM sleep.[72]

Hormones and sleep

Although it seems highly likely that midlife sleep disturbances are triggered by changes in hormones, few studies have been able to demonstrate this directly.[65] A small study of 140 Polish women reported finding that sleep disturbance was linked to high FSH and low estrogen.[73] Other larger studies haven't been able to confirm this, but because of the challenges of studying this subject, it may not mean a link *doesn't* exist. We know that if you have your ovaries surgically removed before you go through menopause, your chances of having significant hot flushing and severe sleep disturbances are at least 80%! Therefore, a sudden loss of your ovarian hormones (primarily estrogen and progesterone) is a major issue for your brain and sleep mechanisms. We also know that taking hormone therapy in this situation improves both hot flushes and poor sleep.[74]

Sleep apnea and hypopnea: Disrupted breathing at night

It seems that as women come into midlife and particularly when transiting from Zone 3 to Zone 4, women start to under-breathe during sleep. In fact, the likelihood that women under-breathe during sleep *increases every year* from Zone 1 to Zone 4.[75] Sleep *apnea* is when you actually *stop* breathing for at least ten seconds at a time during sleep, while sleep *hypopnea* is when your breathing reduces by 50-90% for ten seconds or more during sleep. The longer and more frequent these apnea and hypopnea episodes are, the more severe the problem is.

If you stop breathing or under-breathe at night, your sleep quality will be reduced, you will likely wake up a lot more (even if you don't remember waking), and you will feel a lot more tired during the daytime.[76] Importantly, it causes blood oxygen levels to fall overnight and the health of our body and brain suffers. Given sleep apnea is one of the causes of sleep disturbance in midlife, if you have a persistent sleep disturbance and are chronically tired, you may want to consider getting a sleep study done. Nowadays, sleep studies are very easy to arrange and can even be done in the comfort of your own home.

Your chances of having sleep apnea increase if you:

- snore loudly
- are overweight or obese with body mass index >30
- have diabetes, high blood pressure, or heart problems
- have upper airway problems, chronic sinusitis, or asthma
- have Parkinson's disease or any other neurological condition affecting breathing.

Sleep and dementia

Sleep scientist and expert Professor Matt Walker says in his book *Why Do We Sleep?*[77] that there is now more than enough evidence to suggest that poor sleep is one of the reasons why people develop Alzheimer's disease or dementia.[78] So, as a midlife woman, if you have poor sleep and are soon to be menopausal, you already have one of the risk factors for dementia.[79] Female-brain researcher Dr. Mosconi says, in her book *The XX Brain*,[80] that every 45-year-old woman has a one in five chance of getting dementia, whereas her male counterpart at age 45 has only a one in ten chance.[81] As you may be thinking, women's risk of dementia is an under-studied problem, but thanks to many researchers like Drs Mosconi and Walker, we are now aware of some of the things we can do to decrease our risk of poor-sleep-related cognitive decline if we correct the problem early enough. You can start any time, but obviously the earlier the better.

What is healthy sleep?

Professor Matt Walker's *Why Do We Sleep?* is a very worthwhile read. He explains that while going to bed for eight hours is important, sleeping *well* during those eight hours is more important. When you sleep well, you repeatedly cycle through the three main stages of sleep. The three stages are light sleep, deep sleep, and REM (rapid eye movement) sleep, with each stage lasts between 90-110 minutes. He has shown that during the first half of the night, deep sleep dominates and during the second half of the night, REM sleep dominates. This means that if you are waking in the early hours of the morning, and do not fall asleep again, you may be getting less than ideal REM sleep. On average, 15-20% of your sleep should be deep sleep and 20-25% should be REM sleep and, of all the kinds of sleep, Prof Walker says that deep sleep is the most restorative.

How not enough quality sleep can damage your brain

During sleep, your brain takes a break and the most profound rest it gets is during deep sleep. Only when the brain goes into deep sleep, does it have the ability to 'clean itself'. Like other organs in the body, the brain can suffer from an excess build-up of the day-to-day body-process-related molecules or 'toxins'. Unlike other organs, however, the brain doesn't have the same intricate network of blood and lymphatic vessels to carry out a 'cleaning' process during the day. Instead, the brain uses an intricate network of pathways that involve cerebrospinal fluid and 'glymphatics' that only operate during sleep. These *glymphatics* were only recently discovered in 2012 and are similar to the rest of the body's lymphatic channels, only they are made up of specialized brain cells called glial cells, hence the name 'glymphatics'.[82] This is the brain's brilliant in-built detoxification mechanism that is critical to counteracting the build-up of toxins. It appears that the brain can only activate its glymphatics, and thus cleaning ability, during deep sleep.[83]

If deep sleep is absent or reduced, it appears that the brain's ability to clear its toxins is reduced.[84] When toxins build up excessively, it increases the risk of an excess build-up of 'free radical' molecules that can damage the brain directly and can also promote the accumulation of harmful proteins called *amyloid*. The excess build-up of both free radicals and amyloid over years or decades is linked to the loss of brain cells, and when this loss is severe enough, it can be seen on a CT or MRI brain scan as atrophy. Dementia ensues when there is excessive loss of brain cells or *atrophy*.[85] One of the areas of the brain that is critical for memory, especially short-term memory, is the *hippocampus*. This area of the brain seems to be particularly vulnerable to being damaged by free radicals and excessive levels of the stress hormone called *cortisol*.[86, 87] No doubt, we have all experienced the link between not getting enough sleep the night before and not being able to think or remember things clearly the next day.

Menopause and dementia

We only know of *some* of the possible reasons why women are at higher risk of dementia and one of them is the fact that we go through menopause. Going through an early or sudden menopause (surgical removal of ovaries) in particular, seems to increase dementia risk. The sudden loss of estrogen and other hormones is likely to play a role, but we don't exactly know what it is yet because taking estrogen therapy at menopause doesn't seem to appreciably reverse the increased risk.[88] In fact, there seems to be accelerated loss of brain cells during the *transition* to menopause, well before estrogen and other hormone levels have fallen to low levels. The failure of countless medication clinical trials so far demonstrates just how challenging this disease is and the complexity of the underlying contributors.[89, 90] As a result, more and more clinicians are researching and utilizing a combined approach to increase brain health using lifestyle, diet, and exercise.[91]

Given women's increased risk of dementia and the fact that the brain starts to falter before menopause, perhaps *the* most important time to instigate an effective brain-health program is in Zone 1! One of the top priorities is getting enough quality sleep, and one of the easiest starting points is to exclude or treat hypopnea or apnea if you have it. If you have a sleeping partner, be sure to ask them if you snore. Remember, sleep hypopnea/apnea can cause you to 'wake' throughout the night, even if you don't remember, causing you unexplained daytime sleepiness.[92, 93] Even if you are not concerned about brain health, getting a healthy amount of sleep brings the benefit of reducing many other chronic diseases such as diabetes (that can double your dementia risk), heart disease, and depression.[75, 94] I will cover some of the other ways you can optimize your sleep in **Section Three**.

Abdominal bloating/discomfort and midriff weight gain

Zone 1	Zone 2	Zone 3	Zone 4
♦♦♦	♦♦♦	♦♦	♦

Feeling bloated, swollen, or distended in the abdomen is not a well-recognized midlife symptom, or at least, not one that is usually linked to midlife changes in hormones. In my experience, however, it is a very common complaint and often linked to unexplained midriff weight gain. Some common complaints include 'I feel blown up like a balloon', 'I feel nine months pregnant' or 'I can't take a decent in-breath, because I feel sort of "stuck" under the diaphragm'. In my clinical experience, midlife hormone changes do seem to play a role in these complaints, many of which can be explained by changes in gall bladder function. There is very little scientific research on gall bladder function at any age, let alone during midlife, so it is a largely unexplored area of women's midlife health. Despite the lack of clinical research, gall bladder problems in midlife women are a well-recognized and common problem. In fact, in medical school, we students were taught that if a patient presented with right-sided abdominal pain (the gall bladder sits in the right upper part of your abdomen), we should be suspicious of gall bladder problems.

We were taught to be particularly suspicious if patients fulfilled the 'Four Fs', which were **Female**, **Fat**, **Forty**, and **Flatulent**! Although not a particularly respectful way of putting it, this is how they taught us to remember it. If you develop sludge or stones in the gall bladder, it is called *cholestasis* and *cholelithiasis* respectively.[95] If your gall bladder is very inflamed or infected, it is called *cholecystitis*. Although anyone can get these gall bladder issues at any time, they are *2-3 times more common in women*, especially midlife women. I notice that when reading the few articles available on women and their gall bladders, that women in their forties are presumed to put on weight and thus suffer thicker bile fluid and reduced gall bladder function or emptying (which increases the likelihood of stone formation). Two studies that researched overweight women and their gall bladders however couldn't find a link between putting on weight and gall bladder function.[96] In fact, reduced gall bladder function was shown to be linked to being on a low fat, low-calorie diet, perhaps the opposite of what would be expected.[97]

I believe that it is likely that gall bladder issues in midlife women have *something* to do with changes in hormones. One of the little-known facts about bile and gall bladder function is that high estrogen can *slow* bile production and gall bladder emptying.[98] We know that high estrogen during pregnancy can lead to increased bile sludge and even bile blockages within the liver and gall bladder.[99] We also know that estrogen therapy alters the critical balance between cholesterol, lecithin, and bile acids in bile, and does so in a way that increases the likelihood of gall bladder sludge and stones.[100, 101] You will already have discovered in this book that some midlife women experience a rise in estrogen. So, perhaps it is a rise in estrogen that explains why midlife women are at particular risk of gall bladder issues. With no clinical studies available to confirm or deny this, we can only hypothesize.

In my practice, women who complain of bloating, distension and gall bladder issues, also commonly complain of excess midriff weight gain. My clinical experience tells me that the midriff weight gain in women with gall bladder problems relates to faulty digestion, poor detoxification, poor elimination through the bowels, and excess inflammation. These concepts are challenging to explain and even more challenging to study, but we do know that high estrogen has been found to interfere with the liver enzymes that help eliminate estrogen.[102] We also know that if you are female and have gall stones or have had your gall bladder removed you are more likely to have the 'metabolic syndrome' (MetS).[103] MetS is characterized by abdominal obesity, insulin resistance, high blood pressure, and abnormally high triglycerides and cholesterol.[104] Seeing countless midlife women with bloating complaints and realizing a likely link between this complaint and high estrogen, I developed the Estrogen Clearing Program. As detailed in **Section Three**, this program involves encouraging the clearing of estrogen from the body through optimal liver, gall bladder and bowel function, which is the mainstay of the body's 'clearing house' for estrogen.

Midriff weight gain

Midriff weight gain can be due to an increase in fat tissue around the abdominal organs (*visceral fat*) or outside the abdomen, under the skin (*subcutaneous fat*) or a combination of both. Visceral fat usually makes your trunk look like an 'apple' shape rather than a 'pear' shape and leads to more weight deposition above the navel than below the navel. This is *inflammation*-related weight.

Factors that put you at risk of having an excessive amount of visceral fat include:

- consuming excessive amounts of inflammatory fats and sugars
- suffering from chronic pain or chronic illness
- suffering from chronic stress, or sleep deprivation.

Subcutaneous fat is the kind of fat that you can pick up in your fingers/hands and pull away from the body. This type of fat is deposited more *below* the navel at the front of the abdomen but is also responsible for the loose 'love handles' at the side of the hips and the fat on the thighs. Compared to visceral fat, it is less likely to be related to inflammation, chronic stress or chronic diseases, and more likely to be related to high estrogen.

Other causes of abdominal bloating at midlife

Not all midlife women with abdominal bloating and discomfort have gall bladder problems. If bloating and pain are severe, it may be irritable bowel syndrome (IBS), severe chronic constipation or small intestinal bacterial over-growth (SIBO). Your symptoms may include bloating after meals or at other times, reflux, abdominal pain, alternating loose and hard stools, or intractable constipation or diarrhea. Because of my functional medicine training, I enjoy taking up the challenge where problematic gut symptoms are concerned, because I recognize the importance of optimal gut health in overcoming a lot of women's hormone issues.

Bloating and abdominal discomfort/pain in anyone should be investigated with a thorough clinical history that covers your diet, your bowel motions and any likely or previous food intolerance. I nearly always request a simple plain abdominal X-ray looking for significant constipation because severe constipation is a very common cause of abdominal issues and remains largely unrecognized by the medical profession. I recommend also making a detailed record on the timing of your bloating and abdominal pain, as this can often give clues as to what is causing it. For example, if you bloat for one to three hours *after meals* but not at other times, you may have poor digestion, severe constipation or even SIBO as part of your problem. If you feel bloated at other times and feel worse as the day goes on, you may have high-estrogen-related poor bile flow, especially if you have other symptoms of high estrogen. I also recommend consulting with a healthcare provider that is knowledgeable in IBS and other gut disorders and has experience with food intolerance, clearing constipation (not as easy as it sounds sometimes), improving your digestion and replacing adequate amounts of fiber. More on this in **Section Three**.

IBS and small intestinal bacterial overgrowth

It has been estimated that up to 60% of patients who are diagnosed with IBS have symptoms that are caused by an abnormally high number of bacteria in their small intestine.[105] This is called 'small intestinal bacterial overgrowth' or SIBO. The validity of the diagnostic tests for SIBO have been and are still debated, but most gut experts agree that many patients have SIBO-like symptoms.[106] Patients with SIBO typically report that their abdominal bloating/pain starts within a half hour of eating and lasts for several hours. They usually feel much better in the mornings before eating. If the SIBO is longstanding, however, patients can feel bloated and uncomfortable most of the time. Patients who have flatulence, low gastric acid (due to medication, stress, or illness), chronic gall bladder issues, and longstanding constipation are more at risk of getting SIBO-like symptoms[107] and those who have had it for years often develop other related symptoms including fatigue, poor sleep, rosacea, restless legs, generalized joint pain, painful bladder syndrome and poor cognitive performance or 'brain fog'.[108]

A diagnostic test for SIBO was comprehensively discussed in the 2017 North American Consensus.[109] The validity of this test however has been and still is hotly debated and a recent publication includes an in-depth discussion about why the test should probably not be used to 'diagnose' SIBO.[106] It is likely that many healthcare professionals overuse the SIBO breath test, especially those who are not experienced in taking and translating detailed clinical histories. Most of my colleagues, for example are not versed in exploring SIBO-like symptoms and tend to blanket-diagnose IBS, overlook chronic constipation and go no further than prescribing a FODMAP diet and medications. If you have ongoing abdominal pain and you think you might have symptoms of SIBO, your task is to find a provider who is experienced in taking a detailed clinical history, doesn't rely on expensive testing, and knows to look for possible underlying causes of your symptoms. They should be also experienced in safe dietary interventions, treating constipation, and addressing gut health through the use of anti-inflammatory agents, prebiotic fibers and if needed, gut-active antimicrobial medications.[105, 110] I discuss gut health including digestion, bile flow, gut motility, and the microbiome in **Section Three**.

Breast swelling and swelling of extremities

Zone 1	Zone 2	Zone 3	Zone 4
♦♦♦	♦♦♦	♦♦	♦

A rise in estrogen at midlife may cause you to feel swollen in your breasts, abdomen and extremities. We know that estrogen can be responsible for 'fluid retention' within the body, but there are no studies specifically looking at *where* in the body this fluid retention is most likely to occur.[111] Fluid retention related to heart problems classically involves the feet, ankles and legs and is reduced after lying down and worsened by standing for long periods. This would rarely be a problem in midlife women. Most of the complaints I hear from women in my practice are about swelling involving the ankles, feet, hands, fingers, breasts and abdomen. If you suffer from premenstrual tension (PMT), you may experience this swelling especially during the week prior to a menstrual period.[112]

We don't know the reasons why high estrogen can lead to excess fluid retention in some women, but we do know that both estrogen and progesterone influence 'fluid balance'.[113] It appears that estrogen is more likely to cause fluids to *accumulate* in the body, while progesterone is more likely to reduce it.[114] The actions of both these hormones on body fluid, however, are complex and probably dependent on the action of many other hormones including thyroid hormone and cortisol. Nevertheless, because estrogen can rise a little in midlife and progesterone can fall a little, it is conceivable that fluid balance is tipped towards fluid retention during Zone 1 and Zone 2 and less so after reaching Zone 3 and Zone 4.

Other causes of body swelling: Stress and cortisol

The other hormone that can cause your body to retain fluid and that causes swelling is cortisol. You may already know that cortisol is one of the body's main stress hormones. Cortisol is produced in the adrenal glands and has multiple life-sustaining roles. One of its roles is to regulate salt and water balance in the body and if in excess (through stress or a disorder called Cushing's disease), it can add to fluid retention in the body. High cortisol levels over a long period of time can have a myriad of adverse effects on the body, including loss of muscle and muscle tone, increased abdominal fat (visceral fat), disruption of blood glucose control, thinning of the skin, thinning of the bones, fragility of blood vessels, and lowered immune function. These are the features of Cushing's disease but can be seen to mild degrees in chronically stressed individuals.

If you are having regular or irregular cycles and are experiencing a lot of abdominal or other body part swelling, you can read about the Estrogen Clearing Program and the steps to improve progesterone, especially reducing stress, in **Section Three**. I will also describe the ways in which to detect and manage stress-related elevated cortisol.

Mastalgia, breast soreness

Zone 1	Zone 2	Zone 3	Zone 4
◆◆◆	◆◆◆	◆◆	◆

Mastalgia is the name for soreness in one or both breasts. You may feel it as pain when pressing on the side or the front of your breasts. It can be worse on one side than the other and is usually especially painful to touch around the *side* of the breast near the arm pit. The pain can be there even when you are not pressing the breast, for example when walking or running, or when just wearing a bra. Some women avoid exercise because they find it too painful to wear a support bra let alone exercise vigorously. Mastalgia is a common symptom, affecting more than half of women at some point in their lives. It is severe in at least 10% of women and accounts for about 60% of all visits to the doctor for breast concerns.[115] Given mastalgia affects more than half of all women, you would think it would have been more comprehensively studied. I could only find a handful of population studies that have attempted to find out more about who it affects and *why*.

Having so few clinical studies has meant we still don't know whether or not it is more common in midlife women. Studies from Turkey suggest that it is more common in midlife[116, 117] and those from Korea and Britain suggest that it can get worse from Zone 1 to Zone 3 and that high estrogen is an important factor.[118] Findings from a Welsh breast pain clinic study suggest that mastalgia starts in the early 30s, peaks around age 40, then decreases after 50.[119] Studies from India, Turkey, China, and the UK all seem to suggest that most mastalgia occurs cyclically, becoming most prominent in the last week or two before a menstrual period. Premenstrual mastalgia has been linked to a faster than usual fall in progesterone (relative to estrogen) during the last week of the cycle, but there are too few studies to confirm this.[120] From the little we do know, it is reassuring that mastalgia has not been linked to having breast cancer or getting breast cancer in future.

If you do see your healthcare provider about mastalgia, your investigations should include a breast ultrasound. Also, if you have particularly 'lumpy breasts', you should ask them to request a urine iodine test. If your iodine is low, replacing iodine can sometimes help reduce the pain. In **Section Three**, I will discuss this and other strategies that can also help.

High-estrogen headaches/migraines

Zone 1	Zone 2	Zone 3	Zone 4
♦♦♦	♦♦♦	♦♦	—

If you have suffered from migraine or headaches that occur on a cyclical basis with your menstrual cycle, they may worsen with the increased swings of estrogen at midlife.[121] It is not clear why the natural hormonal fluctuations can trigger headaches or migraine, but while both estrogen and progesterone can play a role, the fluctuations in estrogen seem to be the more likely culprit. Given estrogen peaks can increase a little in Zone 1 and then become more dramatic in Zone 2, these Zones may be the time when headaches worsen. By Zone 4, when estrogen peaks are calming down a lot, the headaches may noticeably settle.

A headache vs. a migraine

The difference between a headache and a migraine is only a matter of severity of symptoms and whether you have other symptoms accompanying it. A headache can be called a *migraine* when it is disabling, greatly impairs routine activities, causes extreme light sensitivity and leads to nausea and sometimes vomiting. Migraine headaches are three times more common and are more severe in women than in men. This gender discrepancy is most likely due to the hormonal fluctuations associated with the menstrual cycle.[122] Up to 45% of women will suffer a migraine headache at some point in their lives. Around 20% of women may have severe recurrent migraine, and one in four of these women also experience a pre-migraine 'aura' that causes loss or change in vision, and sometimes other nerve-type pins-and-needles pain or, rarely, paralysis. If women have auras *frequently*, they should be mindful that they may have an increased risk of stroke.

Although *premenstrual* headache is common, most women who have premenstrual headache suffer from migraine at other times of the cycle as well. Premenstrual migraine is likely triggered by the *drop* in estrogen and progesterone that occurs at the end of the menstrual cycle, but research on this is lacking. What we do know is that a fall in progesterone may lead to a spike in *inflammation* in the body, and the fall in estrogen may lead to adverse changes in neurotransmitters (brain communication molecules) like serotonin.[122] Not all migraine headaches in women are related to hormonal fluctuations, and when there is little relief with usual medications and analgesics, you and your healthcare provider may want to consider other causes, like head and neck muscle tension or upper spine problems, food intolerance, or environmental exposures. I will review these in **Section Three** when I list some of the medications and other solutions that I have found to be effective in my practice.

Aches and pains

Zone 1	Zone 2	Zone 3	Zone 4
♦♦	♦♦♦	♦♦	♦♦♦

Although there seems to be an increase in generalized aching in the joints and/or muscles with increasing age, no symptom study in midlife women has confirmed that these symptoms are linked to changes in hormones.[123] If your aches and pains tend to occur with other symptoms of PMS (premenstrual syndrome), then they can tend to worsen when you are in Zone 1, Zone 2, and less so in Zone 3. If your aches and pains are not PMS-related and become more noticeable in Zone 3 and Zone 4, they may be related to low estrogen or other factors of wear and tear. This is where a full-body maintenance program becomes important. I discuss the need for mobility, relaxation, and strength training as we age in **Section Three**.

Irritability and anxiety

Zone 1	Zone 2	Zone 3	Zone 4
♦♦	♦♦♦	♦♦♦	♦♦♦

Irritability seems to be a very common symptom in midlife women but, again, no symptom study in midlife women has been performed to characterize this further or link it to changes in hormones.[123] In my experience with midlife women, an increase in hormonal fluctuations, can cause them to feel more 'edgy'. I have also found that women in Zone 2 and Zone 3 who are irritable can have symptoms of anxiety, especially when they are dealing with significant life stressors and/or are sleep deprived. Have you noticed that you feel overwhelmed very easily? We can all get anxious about adverse issues in our bodies and our lives, but I find women are a lot *more* likely to feel overwhelmed, teary, and anxious when going through Zone 2 and Zone 3.

Teasing out *why* and *when* midlife women get more irritable or anxious isn't easy in the world of research, because the logistics of studying populations of midlife women and their symptoms can get unimaginably complex. While some studies have found that irritability and anxiety worsen in Zone 4 and beyond, others have found that it is most severe in women who are in Zone 2 and Zone 3.[124, 125] There are so many individual factors influencing how debilitating the anxiety can be, including whether women have suffered anxiety *prior to* midlife.

If you have experienced excessive irritability or anxiety *prior to* Zone 1, I would suggest you take extra care of yourself from your late 40s and actively seek out and implement physical, mental, and emotional support strategies. That way, if you do experience hormonal and mood upheavals, you won't be taken by surprise, and you will be better prepared. If you *haven't* experienced irritability and anxiety before, you may suddenly find yourself a 'different person'. Many women sit in front of me in my office and say, 'It's just not like me to lose it!', or similar. Although many complaints like this have a hormonal basis, other inevitable factors associated with the so called 'midlife crisis' can be playing a role.

Melbourne psychologist Robyn Vickers-Willis says it is very common for women aged between the mid-30s and late 40s to feel confronted by feelings of depression, emptiness, and bewilderment with no idea where it is coming from:

> Our psyche also encourages us to move from having a sense of identity based on how we are conditioned to see ourselves and what others expect of us, to how/who we truly are. This kind of personal 'home-coming' can be very uncomfortable, especially when we haven't honored our desires or wishes when younger. With the mounting commitments and responsibilities in midlife, we can suddenly feel at the end of our tethers, overwhelmed, and feeling a need to 'escape'. Some of us may even turn towards damaging behavior like excessive shopping, exercising to the extreme, or having reckless affairs.[126]

Some of the 'unsettling' feelings and thoughts common to midlife include feeling an overwhelming desire to tackle a goal long forgotten since childhood, suddenly wanting a child or more children, having unexplained depression or listlessness, feeling trapped in a life that isn't wanted, constantly asking, 'Is this all there is?', feeling confronted by mortality and the wish to live a life of greater meaning, and feeling overwhelmed with out-of-control emotions.

Low mood and depression

Zone 1	Zone 2	Zone 3	Zone 4
♦	♦♦	♦♦♦	♦♦♦

Severe depression at midlife is uncommon and when it occurs, it is a serious problem.[127] While the risk of developing severe depression at midlife does *not* seem to increase, some *symptoms* of depression can increase during Zone 2 and Zone 3 compared to Zone 1 and Zone 4.[70, 128] Moreover, if you have experienced depression *prior* to Zone 1, it *may worsen* during Zone 2 and Zone 3.

> **Professor Martha Hickey's Melbourne University research group has found that between Zone 1 and Zone 4:**
>
> - 80% of women have little or no depressive symptoms
> - 9% have a worsening of symptoms
> - 9% get fewer depressive symptoms
> - 2.5% have ongoing severe depression.

Prof Hickey said of their findings, "The slight increase in depressive symptoms during the transition to and after menopause could not have been fully attributed to the fact that they were in the menopause". In other words, factors other than changes in hormones are likely to be contributing to low mood in midlife.[129] Other investigators have examined the role that hormonal changes could play in midlife mood issues by looking into brain chemistry. Their work has shown that there are hormone receptors for estrogen, progesterone, and other hormones all over the brain.[130]

Some hormones appear to regulate inflammation in the brain, with estrogen playing both inflammatory and anti-inflammatory roles.[131] Progesterone also plays a role in regulating inflammation in the brain via the well-known 'GABA' receptors, but it isn't clear whether it is largely inflammatory or anti-inflammatory. There is a vast amount of information to sort through in this area of science, so it may take years for us to make sense of it and draw conclusions. In **Section Three** I will cover some of the basic principles of how to approach mood disorders in midlife, including the use of the Basic Program.

Premenstrual syndrome (PMS)

Zone 1	Zone 2	Zone 3	Zone 4
◆◆	◆◆◆	◆◆◆	—

Premenstrual syndrome (PMS), also known as premenstrual tension (PMT) is a common symptom in women of all ages, with around 30% of women having at least mild symptoms. Between 5-10% of women have a severe form of PMS called PMDD or premenstrual dysphoria disorder.[132] Although it has not been directly studied, PMS seems to become more prominent after Zone 2 and diminish after Zone 4 is reached. This is also true of PMDD, so from Zone 1 to Zone 3, anyone who has suffered from PMDD *in the past* should be watched closely for deterioration so they can be managed urgently if needed.

If you regularly suffer from PMS, you will know a lot about the following symptoms:

- bloating, breast tenderness, swelling of extremities and/or generalized pain
- food cravings (sweet>salty)
- irritability, low mood and/or depression
- mood swings, feeling overwhelmed, emotional, and/or teary
- poor concentration and/or sleep disturbance.

We have already covered many of these PMS symptoms, as many of them can occur in isolation and tend to peak between Zone 1 and Zone 4. Why do so many women get PMS? The short answer is that we don't really know. We do know that there is a genetic susceptibility to PMS, and that there are some yet to be understood factors in the form of stress, diet and lifestyle.[133, 134] We don't know exactly what these factors are yet and whether reducing these factors will reduce the likelihood of getting PMS. Clinical studies suggest that PMS may have something to do with lower estrogen and/or lower progesterone during the luteal phase of the cycle.[112, 135, 136] Other studies have found that a *faster* decline in progesterone at the end of the menstrual cycle makes PMS more likely.[137] In many women however, PMS can start 10-14 days before the menstrual period, well before either estrogen or progesterone start to fall.

Needless to say, we have a long way to go in our understanding of PMS, but I find it a relatively satisfying condition to treat in my practice, because when not accompanied by PMDD, it is responsive to diet, lifestyle, and simple intervention, which I will review in **Section Three**. I will explain why I rarely need to resort to birth control pills or hormone therapy. In the case of PMDD, I make sure all my patients are under the care of a psychiatrist when instigating my diet/lifestyle interventions.

Low libido

Zone 1	Zone 2	Zone 3	Zone 4
♦♦	♦♦	♦♦	♦♦

Between 50% and 80% of midlife and older women are sexually active and, according to a North American study of more than 2,600 women of all ages, midlife and older women don't seem to complain of lower libido any more than younger women.[138] Another study, however, suggests a decrease in sexual activity with age, with weekly sexual activity decreasing from around 52% in women aged 18-44 to around 25% in women aged 65 and older.[139] Some researchers have also found a fall in sexual desire with age, along with an increase in relationship 'issues' which adversely affect sexuality.[140]

Decreased libido at midlife

If we are sexually active at midlife, low libido can be driven by many factors including changes in hormones, unresolved relationships, stagnant partner/marriage dynamics, problems with our physical bodies or self-image, or the fact that we have too many stressors involving our children and/or aging parents. The degree to which hormones play a role is unclear but it is not simply a rise or a fall in estrogen or testosterone, as these two hormones only fall appreciably in Zone 4. Some studies suggest that low libido in women between 35 and 50 has something to do with low testosterone[141] but other studies haven't been able to show an appreciable drop in testosterone between Zone 1 and Zone 3.[142] We know that in normal menstrual cycles, testosterone rises a little immediately before ovulation, but clinical studies to date haven't been detailed enough to detect this small rise in testosterone in relation to changes in libido. We do know that from Zone 4 onwards, combined estrogen and testosterone therapy can be effective in combatting low libido.[143]

Hypoactive sexual desire disorder (HSDD)

Female sexuality is complex and is highly influenced by our relationship satisfaction, our partner's disposition, our own physical health, socio-cultural factors, and our psychological dynamics. In recent years, low sexual functioning and satisfaction has been termed as hypoactive sexual desire disorder or female sexual interest/arousal disorder or HSDD. The definition includes *'absent or diminished feelings of sexual interest or desire, absent sexual thoughts or fantasies, and a lack of responsive desire'*. Motivations for attempting to become sexually aroused are scarce or absent and the lack of interest is considered to be beyond a normative lessening with life cycle and relationship duration.[144] HSDD is thought to affect around 9% of women aged 18-44 and 12% women aged 45-64, but this varies widely between populations and surveys.

HSDD is linked to lower health-related quality of life, lower general happiness and satisfaction with partners, and more frequent negative emotional states.[144] HSDD can affect any of us at some point in our lives and, in women classified as having HSDD, the main contributors include sexual trauma, abuse, poor self-image, dysfunctional relationships, financial and situational stress, poor sleep, excess alcohol, physical illness, fatigue, and even childbirth. If you are interested in finding out whether you may have an issue with sexual desire or arousal, you can do the female sexual function index (FSFI) questionnaire which includes 19 questions within six categories of desire including arousal, lubrication, orgasm, satisfaction, and pain.[145] The questionnaire produces a total score ranging from 2 to 36, with a cut-off of less than 26.5 suggesting sexual dysfunction. Subsequent research has shown that mean scores on the FSFI tend to be lower in midlife and older women compared to younger women.[146]

Increased libido at midlife

Some midlife women in my clinical practice report a heightened libido at midlife. Many of them recognize that this could be part of their 'midlife crisis'. In a report of the findings from the MacArthur Foundation, authors Wethington and Pixley state that "midlife women are turning previous sex roles upside down and are embracing their midlife as a time of powerful renewal. They are now dating and having affairs with younger mates and are enjoying vital, active sex lives over the age of 45."[147] I would hazard a guess that 'overactive' ovaries and bursts of high estrogen at midlife *could* cause some women to express their 'midlife crisis' by having affairs. There aren't any studies yet to confirm or deny this. Heightened feelings of sexuality can also accompany a condition called 'mania', and thanks to a recent study, we now know that women entering the perimenopause may be at increased risk of becoming manic for the first time.[148]

Medications, alcohol, health, fitness, and libido

There are a host of factors that can adversely affect libido including negative self-image, poor self-esteem, unrewarding past sexual experiences, depression, anxiety, or feeling overwhelmed with financial/work/family commitments. Moreover, any kind of physical pain or discomfort can quickly dampen libido, especially if it is causing significant distress. Important examples of libido-dampening symptoms include chronic pelvic pain from endometriosis, adenomyosis or infection causing 'deep dyspareunia' and vaginal dryness or atrophic vaginitis causing 'superficial dyspareunia'. Dyspareunia simply means 'pain with intercourse'. Deep dyspareunia can occur at any age, while superficial dyspareunia is usually confined to women in Zone 3 or Zone 4 and is a result of low estrogen-induced vaginal dryness or atrophy. I will discuss this further in **Section Three**.

Other common causes of low libido are excess alcohol and medications. While alcohol in small amounts can help couples feel more relaxed and 'in the mood', any more than two drinks can dampen proceedings, especially for men who can suffer from alcohol-induced erectile dysfunction. The medications that can reduce libido include antidepressants, particularly SSRIs like citalopram, escitalopram, and fluoxetine. Others include the oral contraceptive birth control pill (OCP), codeine-containing analgesics, seizure medications, beta blockers, and high blood pressure medication. Oral contraceptive pills likely cause a drop in libido by abolishing the normal menstrual cycle, thereby preventing ovulation and the natural surges of estrogen and testosterone.

The OCP can also increase compounds in the blood that bind and inactivate sex hormones (sex hormone binding globulin or SHBG).[149] Some types of OCP are less likely than others to diminish libido, and they include combined OCPs containing drospirenone & ethinyl estradiol or gestodene & ethinyl estradiol.[150] The progestin-only or minipills are less likely to reduce libido, perhaps because they don't abolish ovulation, and instead work to create 'hostile mucus' in the cervix. Libido can also vanish after childbirth because the menstrual cycle is not yet back 'in motion' and will remain out of action until the completion of breastfeeding.

Forgetfulness and poor concentration

Zone 1	Zone 2	Zone 3	Zone 4
♦♦	♦♦	♦♦	♦♦

You may have noticed that once you hit your late 30s and 40s, you tend to forget things, misplace keys, and perhaps at times, don't feel as sharp as usual. I have found these complaints to be quite common in midlife women and although women in all Zones can be affected, I find most improve after Zone 4. A Danish study in midlife women pointed towards persistent midlife forgetfulness as a likely risk factor for getting dementia down the track,[151] and this lines up with other research that tells us that both brain structure and function start to decline *before* Zone 4.[81] We don't know why this happens, whether it happens in all women, or whether it can be prevented. Changes in hormones are likely to play a role, but it isn't clear to what extent. In my practice, I instruct women who complain of memory issues at midlife to start addressing some of the factors that worsen brain health such as poor sleep, stress and poor general health. I also ask them to be particularly watchful concerning any further decline after reaching Zone 4.

We often forget that the brain is part of the *physical* body, and that the health of our body determines the health of our brain. The health of our brain can also have a huge bearing on our mental health. Even before midlife, many of us have experienced feeling foggy in the head from lack of sleep, too much unhealthy food, excess alcohol, or significant stress. While young and healthy, we don't feel these 'insults' as much, but if we develop a chronic medical issue and/or hit midlife or menopause, we may notice that we become a whole lot less tolerant. We can no longer stay up all night, drink a few glasses of wine, then bounce out of bed with a clear head the following morning.

Some of the more common cognitive complaints I hear from midlife women:

- unable to think of the word they want to say
- misplacing their keys or momentarily forgetting where they parked the car
- feeling irritable, anxious, and overwhelmed when faced with multiple complex tasks
- poor sense of direction, especially when following a map to go to a new place
- reading the same line several times before they realize that they're not taking anything in
- feeling unrefreshed after sleep and waking several times through the night.

Looking after your brain and future cognitive capacity should start as early as possible. Once cognitive decline is persistent and measurable, it is likely that significant brain damage has already begun. My initial medical training taught me that memory/cognitive problems were largely irreversible, and that the pharmaceutical approach was superior to anything else. There was no emphasis on optimizing brain health either by optimizing general physical body health or by directly helping the brain. After training in functional medicine however, I now see that improvements in memory and cognitive decline are absolutely possible for many patients through specific and personalized diet and lifestyle strategies.

Reversible factors that could be causing memory and cognitive issues:

- poor gut health
- lack of sleep: difficulty getting to sleep or staying asleep
- excessive stress, trauma, or feeling overwhelmed or 'wired and tired'
- medications for blood pressure, depression, epilepsy, anxiety, asthma, inflammation, etc.
- chronic illness, chronic fatigue, head injuries.

Your gut and your brain

You may have experienced the effect of eating certain foods on your brain or mood. How would you feel for example, after snacking on crisps while sipping on wine, then eating several pieces of delicious pizza, before enjoying a couple of delicious homemade desserts? Perhaps you would feel fine, but perhaps not. Perhaps the following day despite getting loads of sleep, you struggle to concentrate, have headaches, and feel generally unwell or irritable. If this is you, what might have happened? Could your symptoms be a result of your large multi-layered wine-accompanied meal? Yes, absolutely. Alcohol and sugary or processed foods can adversely affect your microbiome and inflame your gut through the production of excess inflammatory 'cytokines'. The excess cytokines can make you 'feel' inflamed in your brain and in your whole body. An inflamed brain in turn can cause you to experience brain fog, irritability and tiredness. Moreover, your symptoms may be worse if you ate something you are 'intolerant' to, you have weak digestion, or your gall bladder isn't working optimally.

Like many midlife women, you may have simply become less tolerant to rich, sugary, processed foods, and less able to handle the 'cytokine storm' that occurs after eating them.[152] We don't know the exact mechanisms yet, but there is a significant connection between your gut and your brain, such that if there is a malfunction in your gut, it may lead to a malfunction in your brain. The relationship between the gut and brain is currently under intense study and has been referred to as the gut-brain axis.[153–155] Although the studies have not yet been done in midlife women specifically, researchers have found that a healthy diet is linked to a healthy mental state.[156, 157] It is likely that this relationship has to do with both the nerves and inflammation. In other words, if the gut is inflamed in any way, it may cause inflammation in the brain, also known as *neuroinflammation*.[158, 159]

Gut problems that may lead to neuroinflammation and foggy thinking:

- poor food choices or regular consumption of 'inflammatory' foods
- upset digestion (eating in a hurry or when stressed)
- inadequate gastric acid, insufficient bile or poor pancreas function
- chronic constipation, inflammatory bowel disease, or disruption to the bowel flora
- gut infections, including diverticulitis and small intestinal bacterial overgrowth.

Gut health was not covered to any great extent in my specialist medical training, so I only learned about its importance after I studied functional medicine and started addressing gut health in my patients. It took some time for me to understand the many ways in which gut *function* can be disturbed and how to apply the myriad management options to individual patients. As an internal medicine specialist, this knowledge has allowed me to solve a much wider array of health issues than I could before. Only recently have I understood gut health to the extent that I can help patients with chronic gut (and brain) problems using individualized medical and nutritional programs. No doubt, there is still a lot to learn.

The nerves in your gut-brain axis

The nerve impulses involved in the gut-brain axis are primarily generated by the *vagus nerve*, its smaller branches, and specialized molecules called *neurotransmitters* (including serotonin, dopamine, norepinephrine and gamma-aminobutyric acid (GABA)). You may have heard of *serotonin*. Serotonin is one of the most important neurotransmitters involved in mood regulation. A little-known fact is that at least 95% of the body's total serotonin is produced in the gut, not the brain. The vagus nerve is responsible for coordinating the digestion, absorption, and elimination of gut contents. Through its vast network of large and small nerves, it carries 'digestion signals' from a centralized system of autonomic nerves to every single area of the gut. As the name implies, this network of nerves functions *automatically*, without conscious input. This part of the nervous system is called the *parasympathetic arm of the autonomic nervous system* and is carried to the gut structures via the vagus nerve. If you ever come across *vagus nerve techniques* or *vagal nerve stimulation techniques*, these are techniques that stimulate the autonomic *rest and digest* functions in the body. Stress is a common cause of dysfunction of the gut and vagus nerve. In fact, whenever you want to improve your gut function, you should always include methods to reduce stress. Stress reduction helps your vagus nerve do its job properly in the gut.[160]

The immune cells in your gut-brain axis
The immune system is what is responsible for inflammation in the body. Having an intact immune system within the gut is critical because it represents the first line of defense against any type of invader organisms that may come into the body via food or drink. If you don't have a properly functioning immune system within your gut, you can be at increased risk of invasive infections called *gastroenteritis*. The gut's immune system relies on nerves, white blood cells and inflammation communication-molecules introduced earlier, called *cytokines*. These cytokines are not only produced in the gut wall, but they are also produced by your gut bacteria, your 'microbiome'. Given your gut microbiome produces cytokines, it follows that the type and amount of cytokines produced is influenced by the kinds of bacteria making up your microbiome. Knowing this paves the way for further research to find out which bacteria tend to lead to healthy cytokines, brain function, and mood and which ones don't.[156]

A 'leaky gut' and neuroinflammation

One of the reasons an *inflamed* gut causes problems is that an inflamed gut can be a 'leaky gut'.[161] Having a leaky gut may sound dramatic, but it doesn't refer to food leaking out into the inside of your body cavities or anything. It refers to an increase in the *permeability* of the inside of the gut wall, whereby more molecules than normal can 'leak' from the gut lumen where food is digested, into the wall of the gut and into the blood vessels within the wall of the gut.[162] If excess molecules leak into the gut wall, they can cause inflammation within the gut wall and this in turn, can cause inflammation in the bloodstream and whole body. A 'leaky' gut is also thought to contribute to unhealthy changes in the blood-brain barrier known as a 'leaky brain' or a leaky blood brain barrier.[163] A leaky brain is what can make you feel fuzzy in the head or headachy and may even underlie some psychiatric disorders.[164, 165]

A 'leaky brain' means that the layer of specialized cells that form a barrier between the bloodstream and the brain is more permeable than what is normal or ideal. A leaky brain therefore would allow more molecules than usual (like *inflammatory cytokines*) to escape from the bloodstream into the brain. If you have a 'leaky brain', your whole brain may become inflamed, and this is referred to as *neuroinflammation*. This is not a good situation, because *neuroinflammation* is linked to poor cognitive function and an increased risk of dementia, stroke, multiple sclerosis, and other neurodegenerative diseases. Neuroinflammation may be a lot more common than we think, and radiology investigator Dr. Wardlaw says "the T2-hyperintense flairs so often seen on MRI scans could be direct evidence of neuroinflammation caused by a breakdown in the blood brain barrier in other words, a 'leaky brain'".[166, 167] When Dr. Wardlaw says *"the T2 hyperintense flairs so often seen on MRI scans"*, she is implying that neuroinflammation is probably a very common problem. In my own practice, I unfortunately often see plenty of women who have both *T2-hyperintense flairs* and suspicious changes in segmental brain volumes, both of which suggest neuroinflammation.[168]

There are many reasons why midlife women could have 'inflamed brains' or neuroinflammation, and it isn't known yet if the hormonal upheavals during this time play a role. Perhaps the underlying causes of neuroinflammation and related brain fog are the same as those underlying hormone-related symptoms. For example, if a patient has a myriad of gut symptoms including a poorly functioning gall bladder, this may lead to both hormone-related and neuroinflammation-related symptoms. Another important cause of neuroinflammation is exposure to a mold-affected or water-damaged home or workplace.[169] Mold illness or mycotoxin illness is becoming increasingly recognized and is characterized by a myriad of symptoms that result from severe inflammation in the body and brain.[170] It has been linked to severe headaches, forgetfulness, poor concentration, mental fatigue, adult-onset anxiety, mast cell activation disorders, fleeting rashes, autoimmunity, and undiagnosed chronic illness. Mycotoxins are the metabolic by-products of molds and become most problematic to human health when the molds are actively growing within the walls, ceilings, or floors of a building.[171] Importantly, mycotoxin illness is *not* an 'allergy' or an 'infection' as such, but rather an *inflammatory* illness. As a result of this and its relatively recent discovery, it is not recognized as an 'illness' by many allergy or infection specialists.

Anxiety, stress and brain health

We know longstanding stress and anxiety can increase the risk of dementia and also reduce cognitive performance in people without dementia.[172] Part of the explanation for this has to do with the stress hormone called cortisol and its adverse effect on the brain, especially the memory center in the brain called the hippocampus. If you are chronically stressed, you will often get persistently high cortisol levels, and these persistently high cortisol levels can damage parts of the hippocampus, causing shrinkage![173] Some of this shrinkage may be reversible, but the longer the cortisol levels remain excessively elevated, the less likely it is reversible.[174] The hippocampus is a part of what is called the *limbic system* which is a curious almond-shaped structure in the center of the brain consisting of the thalamus, hypothalamus, amygdala, hippocampus, and cingulate gyrus. The limbic system plays an important role in survival, notification of danger, emotions, and memories. The amygdala is especially important in generating the 'fight-or-flight' response. Together with the hippocampus, the amygdala also allows us to remember those things that we need to remember for survival.

You may know that the 'fight-or-flight' survival response is governed by what we call the *sympathetic arm of the autonomic nervous system*, that part of the nervous system that controls automatic activities in the body such as breathing, heart pumping, sweating, piloerection, blood pressure, excretion etc. When you are stressed, feel unsafe, or are threatened in any way, the fight-or-flight response is activated by your sympathetic nervous system. This temporarily diverts your attention away from thinking and stops the rest-digest functions in their tracks. As long as the threat remains, the sympathetic drive or fight-or-flight drive is activated. Many of us can recall doing 'silly' things when we are experiencing an acutely stressful or traumatic event, only to recall later after things calm down how silly we were. If your stress, lack of safety, or perceived threat are continuous, your thinking deficits may also be continuous

Chronic stress, chronic illness, anxiety, and trauma can all lead your body to produce an excessive amount of *oxidative stress molecules* which also have the potential to damage your brain.[175] We don't know the whole story about how oxidative stress damages the brain, but we know that our whole brain, not just our hippocampus, is susceptible to its ravages.[176] This is another reason chronic stress may increase your risk of developing Alzheimer's dementia down the track.[177] Excess oxidative stress is highly inflammatory on both the body and brain, and this in turn can worsen anxiety and stress. In this way, oxidative stress can produce a kind of 'feed-forward' cycle which involves stress, inflammation, and anxiety-causing and anxiety-worsening neuroinflammation. This is why I work on reducing whole-body inflammation when addressing health issues that are accompanied by anxiety.

Hopefully, it makes a lot of sense to you now, that learning how to manage stress should be an essential part of optimizing your body and brain health. While most of us work to avoid challenges, this is usually not workable in real life, so we do need to take time out to learn how to manage ourselves and our responses to stress and adversity. I discuss these strategies in **Section Three**, including specific therapies that can calm the 'limbic system' and release trauma.

Hot flushes and night sweats

Zone 1	Zone 2	Zone 3	Zone 4
◆	◆	◆◆	◆◆◆

Hot flushes or hot flashes are the hallmark symptom of menopause. The term *flushes* is used more commonly in the UK and Europe, and *flashes* more commonly in North America. The scientific term used in research is *vasomotor symptoms*, with *'vaso'* meaning blood vessel and *'motor'* referring to the *movement*. Hot flushes are most common in the latter part of Zone 3 and Zone 4, but about one in five women can start experiencing them in Zone 2 and even Zone 1.

In my Ph.D. study, about 20% of my Zone 1 women experienced hot flushes, but they were infrequent, mild, and not bothersome to them at all. In these women, it was most noticeable during the 3-5-day window before their menstrual period.[178] According to one study of African American midlife women, 46% of women experienced hot flushes before Zone 4, compared to 30% in age-matched Caucasian women.[179] In another US-based study, almost 80% of women had experienced daytime or night-time flushing by Zone 4. Between 7-15% of women in Zone 4 suffer *severe* flushes that markedly reduce their quality of life. [180] Information from the SWAN study tells us that women who experience hot flushes have them for an average of about 7-8 years (longer in African American women). If you are a mild flusher, you may only have bothersome flushes for 2-3 years, but if you are a severe flusher, you could have them for ten years or more.[181] Also, if you start flushing while in Zone 1, you will tend to experience them for longer than if you start flushing towards the end of Zone 3 or in Zone 4.

What is it like to have hot flushes?

Typically, when you are having a flush, you feel a sudden and intense sensation of heat coming from deep inside the body, or sometimes just the head, neck, and upper chest area. Prior to the sensation of heat, some women may feel a kind of vague feeling or 'aura' of discomfort, restlessness, anxiety, palpitations, or nausea. Within minutes of feeling the intense sense of heat, a variable degree of flushing of the skin may occur. The flushing usually lasts for 1-10 minutes but can last for up to 15 minutes in some women. Sometimes the flush ends with a sweat and at other times, the skin remains dry, causing what we call a 'dry flush'. Some women get flushing with sweats most of the time, but others may have predominantly dry flushes.

When to expect flushes

Flushes can occur during the day or night, but if you experience flushing during the daytime, you will likely also have night-time flushes, especially if your daytime flushes are severe. It is more common to experience night-time flushes and disrupted sleep without daytime flushes. Flushes at night-time typically occur after waking, but many women describe waking in a pool of sweat after the flush. Here is a common scenario I hear from my patients:

> I often wake up in the middle of the night for no reason, just feeling a bit restless. Then within a minute or so, I start feeling incredibly hot. I have to throw the bed clothes off and try to cool down. Even if I have a fan or air conditioner on, I can't cool down until the flush has subsided 5-10 minutes later. Once it has passed, I can get back to sleep again. It might happen 2-5 times a night.

If you find yourself waking *drenched* in sweat, it is likely you have *already had* a hot flush immediately before waking. If your flushing starts while you are still sleeping, you are not able to initiate body cooling activities (throwing off the covers and fanning, etc.), so your body takes its own action to cool down, and that is to sweat. In this way, it is probably preferable to wake up *before* a hot flush so you can avoid the drenching sweats that disturb your sleep a lot more. Most women who wake at night with hot flushes do get back to sleep between waking, but sometimes the night flushing sets in motion a problematic sleep disturbance.[71] This can then adversely affect the quality and quantity of sleep, and in turn, all aspects of body functioning.

Who gets hot flushes?

The simple answer would be Zone 4 women, because their estrogen and other hormones decline at menopause. It turns out that this is only part of the answer. We know that not all women get flushes at menopause when their estrogen falls, and that most young women who lose their estrogen before age 35 do not suffer from them. Some unlucky women lose their estrogen in their 30s or younger through failure of their ovaries or through breast cancer treatments. Interestingly, these women don't often get hot flushing until their 40s and 50s.[182] In general, if you hit Zone 4 after age 45 or so, hot flushes are more likely than if you arrive at Zone 4 before age 40.[183] Conversely, even if your estrogen levels are within the 'normal range' in Zone 1 and Zone 2, you can start to experience hot flushes.

As I observed in my Ph.D., flushing in Zone 1 and Zone 2 tends to be milder than in Zone 3 and Zone 4 and it seems to occur cyclically just before a period as part of PMS.[184] Perhaps the heightened swings in estrogen along with the slight fall in progesterone play a role. Either way, teasing out the hormonal dynamics underlying hot flushing at midlife represents a logistical nightmare in terms of research, especially given the variability of hormone levels within women, between women, and from cycle to cycle. Thankfully, although we don't have all the answers yet about how hormonal changes cause hot flushes, we have several effective management options available that help relieve severe symptoms in most women.

Hormonal changes and hot flushes

Hot flushes have to do with changes in temperature-regulation. The usual center for controlling your temperature is in the brain in a small area called the hypothalamus. Remember the 'reproductive stage play' in **Section One**, where I explained how the hypothalamus plays the most important role in directing the menstrual cycle 'stage play'? The hypothalamus directs the pituitary below it, which in turn directs the ovaries and influences hormone production. The hypothalamus director not only manages the menstrual cycle stage play, but it also has the enormously complex task of managing other automatic functions including appetite, thirst, fluid balance, and blood pressure.

It makes sense that when the actresses in the stage play (estrogen and progesterone) start to change at midlife, the instructions from both the director and assistant director would adjust as a result.

Figure 9: The multi-tasking hypothalamus

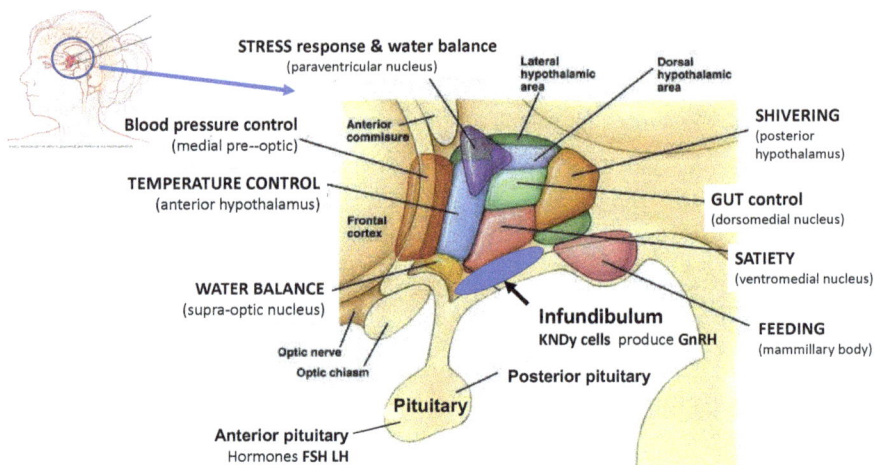

Figure 9 shows a close-up view of the hypothalamus and pituitary in the under-side of the brain. Notice GnRH is produced in a tiny area called the 'infundibular nucleus' at the bottom of the hypothalamus. The nerve cells that produce the GnRH are called KNDy cells. Via its complex language of secretion pulses, GnRH ensures the menstrual cycle functions properly, complete with the peaks and troughs of estrogen, progesterone, and testosterone. The GnRH hormone carries 'signals' to the pituitary gland (via the bloodstream) to tell the pituitary to produce FSH (follicle stimulating hormone). Remember, FSH is the messenger molecule that travels through the bloodstream from the pituitary to the ovary. There, it tells the ovary to produce estrogen and to start another menstrual cycle.

You might remember from **Section One** that both the GnRH and FSH 'signaling' from the brain gets louder when the number of ovarian follicles falls as women progress from Zone 1 through to Zone 4. When the ovary has run out of follicles completely a year or so after menopause, GnRH and FSH levels reach very high levels. Even though the ovary can no longer respond to the FSH (because it has run out of follicles), the GnRH and FSH levels remain high for the rest of your life. An interesting little-known fact is that the KNDy cells within the hypothalamus actually *grow* in size around the time of menopause. It is likely that this is because they are producing such high amounts of GnRH in an effort to get the menstrual cycle back into action. It is thought that the growth of these KNDy cells may somehow influence the nearby temperature control center in the brain and trigger hot flushes. This is a subject of ongoing research and new hot-flush medications targeted at inhibiting KNDy cells have been found to be quite effective at relieving hot flushes. Given their central (brain) mechanism of action however, patients should remain vigilant about possible adverse side effects.[185-187]

Do falling levels of progesterone have anything to do with getting hot flushes?

We don't know, but falling progesterone levels may contribute to hot flushes in women in Zone 1 and Zone 2 when they are unlikely to be experiencing a fall in estrogen. We know that progesterone causes around a ½-degree (Celsius) *rise* in temperature during the luteal phase, a feature of progesterone that allows basal body temperature to be used to detect ovulation.[188] What we don't know is whether its role in temperature regulation influences hot flushing. Progesterone therapy can reduce night sweats, particularly when taken as a tablet before bed.[189] More on this in **Section Three**.

Factors that influence severity of hot flushes

Compared to Caucasian and Hispanic women, women who have African genetics are for some reason more susceptible to severe and frequent hot flushes before and after Zone 4, while Asian women seem to be less susceptible.[190] Although not the rule, it appears that if your mother or aunt or grandmother has severe flushes, then you are more likely to get them as well.[191] The level of fitness doesn't seem to have anything to do with risk of having flushes, although they are more likely in obese women.[192] Other individual factors such as lifestyle, smoking, stress, and sleep also play a role and you are more likely to get severe hot flushes if you have a long history of depression or have had longstanding PMS. Less education, hysterectomy, ovary resection, and chemotherapy are also linked to more severe hot flushes.

You are *more* likely to have severe hot flushes if you:

- have a first degree relative who had severe hot flushes
- currently smoke or have smoked heavily in the past
- have had your ovaries removed in midlife
- are severely overweight or obese (body mass index 30 or over)
- don't have a higher education
- have predominantly African genetics.

You are *less* likely to have severe hot flushes if you:

- are more mindful or practice mindful techniques
- use methods like cognitive behavioral therapy or meditation
- use estrogen and/or progesterone therapy after menopause
- have predominantly Asian genetics.

Alcohol consumption and hot flushes

A number of studies have looked at whether there is a link between the alcohol you consume and hot flushes. Two studies showed that if you are in Zone 2 or beyond and consume 1-5 alcoholic drinks per week, you are *less likely* to experience hot flushes than if you *don't* drink at all.[193, 194] Another study showed that if you are in Zone 1 and consume 3-8 drinks per week, you are *more likely* to get hot flushes than if you don't drink.[195] Although a clear relationship is not yet evident, it is likely that alcohol probably doesn't prevent or cause hot flushes. Some forms of alcohol, however, like red wine, can trigger a flush in some people, particularly if they are already flushers.

It is worth mentioning here that alcohol consumption is linked to risk of breast cancer, with as few as 3-6 drinks a week significantly increasing your risk.[196] In a review of 15 alcohol and breast cancer studies, the authors concluded: 'All levels of evidence showed that alcohol consumption is linked to the risk of breast cancer in a dose-dependent manner, even at low levels of consumption'. In other words, the more alcohol consumed the higher the risk.[197] We don't know exactly why alcohol consumption increases risk, but it could have something to do with upsetting the normal elimination of estrogen from the body via the liver. Drinking alcohol doesn't seem to raise blood levels of estrogen or progesterone, but it has been shown to raise the *excretion* of certain estrogen breakdown products in the urine.[198, 199] The significance of the changes in estrogen breakdown products remains unclear but the take-home message is that alcohol should be enjoyed on occasions and not drunk habitually or daily. While there seem to be cardio-vascular benefits from alcohol, this doesn't appear to require habitual or daily intake.[200]

Stress and hot flushes

Stress appears to be both a *trigger* for hot flushes, and *a consequence* of having severe hot flushes. We don't know however whether being stressed would convert you from being a non-flusher to a flusher. Life stressors tend to accumulate with age and, as midlife women, our lives are often full of concerns. Our worries may include diminishing fitness/strength, aging and loss of youth, loss of partners, increased work-related responsibilities, aging/ailing parents, etc. Whereas some of us sail through our challenges, some of us get increasingly stressed and anxious. The *way* we handle what life presents to us is key to determining whether we become stressed or not. Studies suggest that our 'perceived stress' is what is linked to the severity of hot flushes, and this has been confirmed in many studies.[201]

If you have lower perceived stress and are of a more mindful disposition, you are less likely to have severe hot flushes.[202] Having a positive outlook on life (and 'emotional intelligence') also reduces your likelihood of having more bothersome hot flushes and increases your chances of having a generally positive experience at menopause.[203] The long-running SWAN study also showed a clear and strong link between perceived stress and severity or persistence of hot flushes. Although we don't fully understand the link between stress and severe hot flushes, it probably has something to do with the actions of the stress hormones cortisol and adrenalin. Even brief elevations of these stress hormones at the wrong time could have a dramatic effect on your autonomic nervous system, which in turn can have a dramatic effect on the function of your blood vessels.

The autonomic nervous system and hot flushes

As its name implies, the autonomic nervous system is *automatic* and can function without conscious input. There are two arms of the system that act in balance with each other: the previously discussed survival 'fight-or-flight' aspect (sympathetic nervous system) and the more relaxed 'rest and digest' aspect (parasympathetic nervous system). The hormones, functions and actions of the sympathetic and parasympathetic nervous system are listed below:

Table 3: The sympathetic and parasympathetic nervous systems

Autonomic Nervous System	Functions	Hormones involved
Sympathetic	Fight and Flight	Adrenalin Cortisol
	Actions	
	• Constricts blood vessels • Increases heart rate and blood pressure • Dilates pupils • Causes goose bumps • Increases sweating • Is stimulating	

	Functions	Hormones Involved
Parasympathetic	Rest and Digest	Acetylcholine Prolactin Oxytocin
	Actions	
	• Causes your intestines to digest food • Allows bladder and bowel to empty • Governs sexual arousal • Is relaxing • Slows heart rate • Causes saliva and digestive enzymes to flow • Activates secretion from numerous glands	

Both parts of the system are necessary for survival, and each can override the other when necessary. The sympathetic can override the parasympathetic nervous system in order to get out of or manage an emergency situation. You simply wouldn't want to be using any energy digesting a meal when you're hanging on for life on a rock-face or being chased by an angry bull. The parasympathetic nervous system can override the sympathetic nervous system when you are relaxing after a meal or practicing meditation or relaxation. If you are chronically stressed, your sympathetic system can constantly override your parasympathetic system to the degree that it can block or greatly weaken your digestion and adversely affect other rest and digest bodily functions.[204]

Being in sympathetic overdrive can increase hot flush severity through:

- reducing your ability to tolerate pain and discomfort
- reducing your ability to relax
- increasing blood vessel reactivity
- increasing the likelihood that a flush will be triggered.

Heart rate variability training: A way to reduce body stress

I didn't know it at the time, but when I was managing my endometriosis using 'vata-calming' strategies I was, in effect, reducing my sympathetic drive and encouraging my rest and digest functions. There are many ways to reduce sympathetic overdrive, and one of the most well-studied methods is heart rate variability or HRV training.[205] The pattern of your heart rate can tell you whether you are, and to what degree you are, in sympathetic overdrive. When *not* in sympathetic overdrive and your rest and digest functioning is healthy, your heart rate will increase slightly during your in-breath and decrease during your out-breath. Your HRV is a measure of the variation in your heart rate between your in-breath (heart rate increases) and your out-breath (heart rate should decrease) within a specific time frame. The higher the heart rate variability (high HRV) between your in-breath and out-breath, the less likely you are in sympathetic overdrive.

Having a *low* HRV is linked to chronic stress, poor sleep, illness, chronic fatigue states, anxiety, and trauma. If you are chronically stressed, are overweight *and* have severe hot flushes, it is like a triple whammy, and your overall risk of chronic disease in general can greatly increase.[206-208] HRV training is very simple, doesn't require any specific devices and can be done in your own home. Although not a necessity, I find the apps and devices that monitor HRV incredibly helpful in conveying when HRV practice is needed most.

Treating hot flushes

Hot flushes should be treated if they are bothersome, and especially if they are causing you sleeplessness and stress. Not only are hot flushes in themselves a marker of cardiovascular disease risk, but they can worsen already disturbed sleep which increases your risk of chronic diseases. I will cover the approaches that you can take to help manage hot flushes and other related issues, like disturbed sleep and mood problems, in **Section Three**.

Having ongoing untreated hot flushes could result in you:

- being in sympathetic overdrive most of the time
- increasing your risk of getting early heart disease or stroke
- getting high blood pressure needing medical treatment

- having high levels of cholesterol and fats in the blood needing medical treatment
- getting insulin resistance, a pre-diabetic state or diabetes
- having disturbed, poor-quality sleep
- getting depressed and/or anxious.

Vaginal dryness, vaginal atrophy, and vaginal pain

Zone 1	Zone 2	Zone 3	Zone 4
—	—	◆	◆◆◆

Vaginal dryness can occur in all the Zones, but it becomes more common in Zone 3 and Zone 4. It is usually noticed during sexual intercourse as a burning or sharp pain around the opening of the vagina and/or the inside of the vagina. When severe, it can make sexual intercourse impossible. The pain results from abnormal friction in and around the vagina during intercourse. Normally the vagina is lined with thick, moist and elastic 'mucous membranes', but with vaginal dryness or atrophy, the elasticity and moisture are lost. This loss occurs because of a fall in estrogen, hence why it is most common in Zone 4. Without estrogen, the mucous membranes lose the 'signal' to maintain their mucus production. This causes a dry vagina. If a dry vagina is left untreated for years to decades, the vaginal mucous membranes become thin and the muscles in and around the vagina lose their strength and bulk. This is called *vaginal atrophy* or *atrophic vulvovaginitis*. This condition leads to shrinkage of the vaginal wall, and the muscles that support the vagina, bladder, urethra, and the other pelvic structures. Related symptoms include burning or pain with urination, urine incontinence and, if severe, vaginal or rectal prolapse. Atrophic vaginitis is not uncommon but only develops if vaginal dryness is left untreated.

Recurrent cystitis, bacterial vaginosis and vaginal thrush

Zone 1	Zone 2	Zone 3	Zone 4
—	—	◆	◆◆◆

Having vaginal dryness can increase your risk of recurrent urinary tract infections (recurrent cystitis), vaginal infections (bacterial vaginosis) and vaginal thrush. This increased risk has to do with the loss of healthy mucous membranes in and around the vagina. This loss leads to a breakdown of the natural 'barrier' to invading organisms including harmful bacteria and candida. The openings to both the vagina and bladder sit right next to the opening to the bowel, so these areas are always teeming with potential invader organisms from the bowel. If the vaginal and perineal mucous membranes are not healthy, they may *not* be forming an effective barrier against these potentially harmful organisms.

You may be at increased risk for recurrent cystitis, vaginosis and vaginal thrush if your resident vaginal and bowel flora are not healthy. Recurrent cystitis is common in Zone 4 especially when there is vaginal dryness of atrophy. Vaginosis and vaginal thrush on the other hand, are not unique to midlife or menopause, even though in some women, low estrogen is a trigger. Estrogen not only keeps the lining of the vagina healthy, but it also stimulates the mucus to produce *glycogen*. Glycogen is the main food source for the healthy resident bacteria, called lactobacillus. If estrogen falls, your ability to secrete glycogen-rich mucus falls and this in turn, can cause the number of healthy resident lactobacillus to fall. The less resident lactobacillus in your vaginal flora, the more likely invader organisms can come in and take over.

The management of recurrent cystitis, vaginosis and vaginal thrush is most effective when using a combination of approaches. The first is to treat the invading bacteria or thrush, the second is to improve mucous membrane health and the third is to increase the health and diversity of the vaginal and bowel flora. This is especially important if you need repeated courses of antibiotics for cystitis, because repeated courses can eventually make matters worse by disrupting the healthy bacteria in the vagina and bowel. While treating recurrent cystitis with repeated course of antibiotics can *increase* the likelihood of future bouts of cystitis, in most cases, it must still be treated with antibiotics. Cystitis is a very common cause of serious blood infections that may require hospitalization and intravenous antibiotics. I will cover the ways you can address your gut health to combat recurrent vaginal infections and cystitis in **Section Three**.

Recurrent cystitis, vaginosis and vaginal thrush are linked to:

- loss of the healthy mucous membranes in and around the vagina
- loss of the protective vaginal flora (resident bacteria), especially lactobacillus
- excess invasive-type bacteria in the bowel.

Preventing recurrent cystitis, vaginosis and vaginal thrush is about:

- treating the invading bacteria or thrush
- improving the health of the mucous membranes in and the around the vagina
- improving vaginal and bowel flora.

Painful bladder syndrome

Zone 1	Zone 2	Zone 3	Zone 4
◆	◆	◆	◆

If you need to urinate frequently (on the hour or every two hours) and have constant pain in the bladder and/or pelvis, you may have an uncommon condition called *bladder pain syndrome (BPS)* or, as it has been previously termed, *interstitial cystitis*. Symptoms include frequent urination during the day and night and severe pelvic pain, especially during urination, that is poorly responsive to analgesic medication.

BPS can occur in women at all ages, but it most commonly starts in the mid-30s. It was previously thought to be most common in menopause, but recent research suggests that this isn't the case.[209] The underlying cause remains unclear, but some believe it can occur due to a build-up of oxalate crystals in the bladder. The oxalate crystals cause intense inflammation, and this leads to pain. The crystals can also cause recurrent infections because bacteria can 'hide out' within the crevices of these crystals that can become embedded within the inside wall of the bladder. Others believe it is caused by excessive and overactive *mast cells* within the bladder wall.[210]

Mast cell activation syndrome as a cause of bladder pain

When mast cells are over-activated in the body, it can lead to, or be a part of a *mast cell activation disorder*. Mast cell activation syndrome is a recently recognized disorder and refers to a systemic condition where patients suffer from all manner of inflammatory and allergic symptoms, including fleeting skin rashes, intermittent flushing, pain, and postural orthostatic tachycardia, or POTS. It can also contribute to the often-unbearable pain in chronic fatigue, fibromyalgia and reflex sympathetic dystrophy, also known as chronic regional pain syndrome (CRPS). Not only can overactive mast cells cause pain syndromes like painful bladder syndrome, but they can also cause severe vaginal pain (vulvodynia) and excessive menstrual bleeding. New York physician Dr. Afrin has published several reports about the successful treatment of heavy menstrual bleeding with anti-mast cell therapies given orally and/or vaginally.[211] Prominent mast cell researcher Dr. Theo Theoharides at Tufts University School of Medicine says, 'Mast cell disorders are complex and are implicated in many adult disorders. There appear to be an increasing amount of mast cell triggers in our modern lives, more than ever before.'[212]

Bone loss and osteoporosis

Zone 1	Zone 2	Zone 3	Zone 4
—	♦	♦♦	♦♦♦

The link between menopause and bone loss is well known, but what is not commonly known is that bone loss seems to start *before* menopause. Research suggests that bone density can start to decline in Zone 2. It has been observed to decline faster again in Zone 3 and for about two years after Zone 4. Bone loss continues after this time, but at a slower rate.[213] If bone loss is rapid, you can end up with thin bones, a condition known as *osteoporosis*. Given that bone loss occurs before menopause, factors other than loss of estrogen are likely to be playing a role. Some researchers have proposed that the midlife rise in FSH could play a role, while others propose that it may be the fall in progesterone.[214] FSH is known to act on bone cells to help bone remodeling and progesterone helps lay down new bone.[215] We know that giving estrogen can prevent bone loss when given in Zone 3 and Zone 4 women, but we don't know whether giving progesterone would have a similar effect.

A *high* bone mass in your 20s or 30s is linked to *less* osteoporosis later in life, especially if you keep active from your 40s and beyond. Resistance exercises have been shown to be more effective in this regard than aerobic exercises like running or jogging. You may be surprised to hear that swimming is a form of resistance exercise, even though you are not weight-bearing. Swimming is like using weights but in the water.

You are more likely to suffer from greater bone loss at midlife if you:

- have a close relative with osteoporosis
- have been inactive most of your life
- have been sedentary for several years before menopause
- are Caucasian and a slight build
- have inflammatory arthritis
- smoke or have smoked heavily in the past
- have taken courses of corticosteroid medication for either asthma or other medical conditions (prednisolone, cortisone and inhaled steroids).

Being overweight affects your bones

Being overweight or obese can have variable effects on your bones. If you are obese and have had longstanding irregular menstrual cycles (leading to less ovulation than normal), you may be predisposed to more bone loss prior to and during menopause. If you are obese, have regular cycles, are in good health and are continually active, you may be spared of any bone loss prior to and during menopause. This is because estrogen is produced in fat tissue, and this estrogen can help protect your bones especially after menopause. There are, however, other health risks involved in being overweight or obese, such as hormone-dependent cancers like breast cancer.[216]

Factors linked to excess bone loss or reduced peak bone mass:

- being chronically unwell and confined to bed for prolonged periods
- having diabetes
- having longstanding chronic inflammation or autoimmune disease
- having present or past low vitamin D level
- having longstanding irritable bowel symptoms or iron deficiency of unknown cause
- eating fast, packaged, take-out meals and/or deep-fried/sugary foods
- eating a diet devoid of fresh vegetables, nuts, seeds, and calcium-rich foods.

Vitamin D and bone

One of the most important nutrients for bone health is vitamin D. The first thing to understand is that vitamin D is not really a vitamin. It is more correctly described as a hormone. Among the many roles vitamin D plays in the body is the regulation of the intake (absorption from the gut), excretion, and balance of both calcium and phosphorous. Our liver and kidneys produce the inactive vitamin D precursor molecules, and these molecules are changed to the active form of Vitamin D (also called Vitamin D3) in the skin when exposed to sunlight. This critical last step conversion is reduced or abolished if you use sunscreen and is also adversely affected by advancing age. The older we get, the less efficient we are at getting an optimal supply of vitamin D from our skin when exposed to the sun.

Vitamin D the super-hormone

Vitamin D plays an important role in the regulation of blood glucose via its effect on the hormone called insulin. It is also critical for healthy immune function, and helps protect you from autoimmune conditions, inflammatory diseases, and disorders of mood and emotion. It reduces oxidative stress and plays an important role in neuro-protection and neuro-regeneration. Low vitamin D has been linked to multiple sclerosis and several neurodegenerative diseases, such as amyotrophic lateral sclerosis, Parkinson's disease, and Alzheimer's disease. Low vitamin D has also been linked to poor immune cell (white blood cell) function and an increased risk of serious outcomes in viral infections.[217]

For reasons that are not clear, vitamin D deficiency appears to be on the increase. So, even if you think you get enough sun exposure, if you have an autoimmune disorder, diabetes, thyroid issues, or recurrent viral infections, you should get your vitamin D levels checked. Midlife is also an ideal time to check your vitamin D level, and to optimize your exercise and diet to ensure you are doing your best to keep your bones strong and healthy. Magnesium, boron, and vitamin K2 are also important nutrients for healthy bones and will be discussed in **Section Three**.

Midlife changes in the immune system, the thyroid and autoimmunity

Features of hormonal-related changes in the immune system:

- fleeting skin itching or sensations of 'crawling under the skin'
- skin rashes or flushing
- headaches
- fatigue and tiredness
- auto-immune conditions including thyroid autoimmunity.

Between 15-30% of perimenopausal women have an *under*-functioning thyroid, where they experience symptoms of an *under*-active thyroid (*hypo*thyroidism) without clear changes in their thyroid function on blood testing. [218-220] Another 5-10% of perimenopausal women suffer from an *over*-active thyroid (*hyper*thyroidism).[221] Both conditions are linked to being female, but only an *under*-active thyroid is linked to midlife or perimenopause, with little clarity about how midlife hormone changes can trigger it.[222] Both *under*-active and *over*-active thyroid issues are often caused by 'autoimmune' disorders, and these are called Hashimoto's thyroiditis and Grave's disease respectively. An autoimmune disorder occurs when your own immune system produces antibodies that react with a part of your body, and in the case of Hashimoto's and Grave's, your own antibodies attack your thyroid. In Hashimoto's, the antibodies mostly lead to an *under*-active thyroid and in Grave's, the antibodies cause an over-active thyroid.

Interestingly, just over 10% of the population produce thyroid antibodies that are detectable on routine blood testing, and at least 27% of women and 7% of men have evidence of Hashimoto's thyroiditis when their thyroid is examined under a microscope.[223] The two antibodies normally found in Hashimoto's are called *anti-peroxidase* and *anti-thyroglobulin* antibodies. It isn't known why so many people produce thyroid antibodies, but a combination of genetic susceptibility, hormonal changes,[224] environmental/dietary factors, and what is called immunological tolerance are all likely to play a role.[225] The thyroid antibodies attack the thyroid and cause inflammatory cells to build up within the thyroid gland leading to the eventual destruction of thyroid-producing tissue.[36] In about 20% of Hashimoto's patients, other organ specific antibodies are produced as well. Many studies have also demonstrated that having Hashimoto's means you may have an increased risk of cancers of the thyroid, breast, lung, and urogenital system, leukemia and lymphoma.[226]

Whenever a patient has symptoms of an *under*-active thyroid, I routinely check for thyroid antibodies, other kinds of autoantibodies, in addition to blood selenium and urine iodine. A deficiency in selenium or iodine is common and can lead to an *under*-active thyroid.[227] Iodine deficiency can also lead to a lumpy thyroid gland or 'goiter'. A goiter is usually easy to see and feel on the front of your neck just above the space between your collar bones. Thyroid cancer doesn't usually cause a goiter, however if you have *any* thyroid lumps, see your health provider about arranging some tests to exclude thyroid cancer.

These tests normally involve a thyroid ultrasound, and if a lump or lumps are verified on the ultrasound, a further thyroid scan using nuclear medicine technologies is recommended.

In my practice, I see many women with *under*-active thyroid, and while it is theoretically easy to treat with thyroid-replacement medication, many women have a challenging time getting symptom relief without also addressing whole-body health. Because Hashimoto's is essentially an inflammatory disorder, I manage *under*-active thyroid patients using both medication and anti-inflammatory diet and lifestyle strategies. I will cover this and more in **Section Three**.

Before moving on to **Section Three**, you may find it helpful to review the FAQs in Table 4 below.

Table 4: Frequently asked questions about your hormones, ovulation, and menstrual cycle

Question	Answer
When are you likely to be ovulating normally?	At any age with a normal cycle length e.g., 24-32 days between menstrual periods
When is your ovulation likely to be faulty with 'cycle stacking'?	When you have a short cycle length of 14-19 days, i.e., when you are bleeding 'twice a month'
When are you likely to have *higher* than normal *estrogen* levels	When you have reached Zone 2 or Zone 3 and are experiencing alternating long and short menstrual cycles
When are you likely to have *lower* than normal *estrogen* levels	In Zone 4 and getting hot flushes and night-time sweats and/or vaginal dryness
When might you have *lower* than normal *progesterone* levels	Age 35 or older with regular or irregular cycles
When are you likely to have *low* *progesterone* levels	In Zone 4 and also in Zone 3 or Zone 2 when you have an irregular cycle length or long cycles of >60 days

The Solutions

The Basic Program
The Estrogen Clearing Program
The Progesterone Support Program

Targeted Solutions (1)
Targeted Solutions (2)
Targeted Solutions (3)

S ection Three contains the **To Do's** that include detailed diet and lifestyle strategies that are tailored to your Zone, your symptoms and your individual needs. I intend that these strategies will inspire you to take charge of your current and future health and allow you to work with whatever medical or surgical intervention that your own healthcare provider advises.

The fundamental basis or starting point for achieving optimal health is the *Basic Program* (**BP**). I recommend this for *all* women in all Zones in addition to other programs that are required for your Zone and your specific symptoms. These other programs include Hormone Support Programs (**ECP, PS,** or **HT**) and Targeted Solutions (**TS**). Please use the index in **Table 5** to locate your program

The **solutions roadmap** below the table (**Figure 10**) shows you how to determine which Hormone Support Program and Targeted Solution would suit you best. I suggest carefully reading the entirety of the Basic Program first. You can then skip to whichever Hormone Support Program and/or Targeted Solution that you have determined suits you.

Figure 10: Your Roadmap according to the Zones

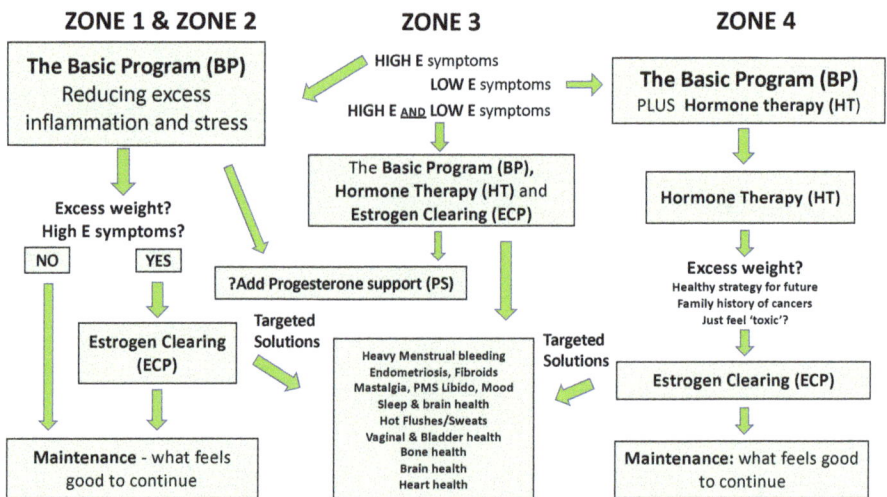

<small>Dr Georgina Hale, MD, Ph.D.</small>

Pointers for the solutions roadmap – Figure 10:

At the top of **Figure 10**, locate your Zone and follow the downward arrows to determine the steps that are relevant to you. If you don't have menstrual periods to help you work out what Zone you're in, you can get an idea of your Zone by using the list of symptoms in **Table 6** on **page 103-104**. Your symptoms can give you some clues as to which Zone you may be in, and the matching Hormone Program or Targeted Solution recommended for that symptom. As you can see from the roadmap, all Zones start with the Basic Program, which can be used alone for general health maintenance even without adding any other programs or solutions.

The **Progesterone Support** and **Hormone Therapy Programs** and **Targeted Solutions** can be started at the same time as the **Basic Program**, but if there is no urgency, I recommend taking 1-2 months to get acquainted with the Basic Program prior to adding other programs.

Women in Zone 3 are more likely than any other Zone to have a combination of high and *low* estrogen symptoms, so if you're in Zone 3, use your knowledge from **Section Two** and **Table 6** to determine whether your symptoms suggest high or low estrogen, or both.

Women in Zones 1, 2, and 3 can also use **Table 6** to discern whether Progesterone Support (PS) could be helpful as part of your program.

Table 5: Index for your Solutions

Table 6: Using your symptoms to determine your Zone

Symptom	Zone				Solution
	1	2	3	4	
Menstrual bleeding and pain problems					
Heavy bleeding with regular periods	♦♦♦	♦♦	♦	—	**BP** with **ECP** and sometimes **PS**
Erratic frequent periods	—	♦♦♦	♦♦	—	**BP** with **ECP** and **PS**
Endometriosis or adenomyosis	♦	♦	♦	♦	**BP** with extra attention to stress reduction and possibly **PS**
Uterine fibroids	♦♦	♦♦♦	♦♦♦	♦	**BP** with **ECP**
Physical body symptoms (persistent or cyclical as part of PMS)					
Abdominal bloating/ discomfort, midriff weight gain	♦♦♦	♦♦♦	♦♦	♦	**BP** with **ECP** and possibly **PS** with **TS**
Mastalgia, breast soreness	♦♦♦	♦♦♦	♦♦	♦	**BP** with **PS** and **ECP** (see also **TS** for mastalgia)
Swelling hands, feet	♦♦♦	♦♦♦	♦♦	♦	**BP** with **ECP** and possibly **PS**
Aches and pains	♦♦	♦♦	♦♦	♦♦♦	**BP** with **ECP** and/or **PS** if needed
High estrogen headache and migraine	♦♦♦	♦♦♦	♦♦	—	**BP** with **ECP**
Mental and cognitive symptoms (persistent or cyclical as part of PMS)					
Irritability and anxiety	♦♦	♦♦♦	♦♦♦	♦♦	**BP** with **PS** and **HT** if Zone 3 or 4
Low mood and depression	♦	♦♦	♦♦♦	♦♦♦	**BP** with **PS** and **HT** if Zone 3 or 4
Low libido (Zone 1 and 2)	♦♦	♦♦	♦♦	♦♦	**BP** with **PS** and **TS**
Low libido (Zone 3 and 4)	♦♦	♦♦	♦♦	♦♦	**BP** with **HT** and **TS**
Forgetfulness and poor concentration	♦♦	♦♦	♦♦	♦♦♦	**BP** with **PS** or **HT** and **TS**
Broken disturbed sleep	♦♦	♦♦	♦♦♦	♦♦♦	**BP** with **PS** and **TS**
Flushing, vaginitis, headaches and sleep problems in menopause (Zone 4)					
Hot flushes and night sweats	♦	♦	♦♦	♦♦♦	**BP** with **HT**; consider **ECP** and **TS**

Symptom	Zone				Solution
	1	2	3	4	
Vaginal dryness and vaginal pain	—	—	◆	◆◆◆	**HT** and/or **TS** for vaginal health
Recurrent cystitis and vaginal infections	—	—	◆	◆◆◆	**HT** and/or **TS** for vaginal health and probiotics
Low estrogen headache and migraine	◆	◆	◆	◆◆◆	**BP** with **HT** and **ECP**
Disturbed sleep	◆◆	◆◆	◆◆◆	◆◆◆	**BP** with **HT** and **PS** and **TS**
Miscellaneous					
Bladder pain syndrome	◆	◆	◆	◆	**HT** or **TS** for vaginal health and painful bladder
Brain health	—	—	◆	◆	**BP** with **TS** for sleep with emphasis on stress reduction and exercise
Heart health	—	—	◆	◆	**BP** with **TS** for heart health with emphasis on stress reduction
Bone loss and osteoporosis	—	◆	◆◆	◆◆◆	**BP** with **HT** and **TS** for bone health including weight-bearing exercise

KEY: BP = The Basic Program; **ECP** = Estrogen Clearing Program; **PS** = The Progesterone Support Program; **HT** = Hormone Therapy with estrogen with or without progesterone; **TS** = targeted solution; **PMS** = premenstrual syndrome

SECTION THREE

The Solutions

The Basic Program

The Basic Program:
Optimal health through reducing inflammation

The fundamental aim of the Basic Program is to optimize health naturally through the elimination or reduction of *excess inflammation* in the body. Inflammation has the potential to cause and perpetuate chronic disease, especially if we regularly consume a highly processed western diet and are largely sedentary. Urban living can add toxic levels of stress when we are swept up by a financially-driven competitive society that leaves a lot of the basic mental and spiritual needs behind.[228] Many of us now realize that it is up to the everyday person to restore sanity and humanity to our lives and communities, and this can only happen if we pay attention to and upgrade our own health and quality of life.

There are no medications involved in the Basic Program, only actions to take in your kitchen and your daily routine. Even if you are struggling with significant depression, anxiety, and/or situational stress, the Basic Program could be the game changer you have been looking for. If, after reading through what is involved in the Basic Program, you think it would be too challenging for you right now, I would advise delaying it until you feel ready. When explaining the features of the program, I will help you prioritize the steps in terms of which ones would be the most important to start first. In the meantime, you could simply focus on understanding the concepts of the program and set up a support network of people and props around you to help you start it then keep on track. Self-care and attention to your unique circumstances are the keys to being able to choose the best way forward.

Your body usually becomes *inflamed* when:

- you are fighting an infection or recovering from an accidental or surgical wound
- your body is over-reacting to a food or environmental toxin
- you are extremely stressed or traumatized.

How do you test for inflammation?

If you don't have an inflammatory illness or an active infection like a virus or an infected wound, testing your body for inflammation can turn up a blank, especially using routine measurements of inflammatory markers like CRP (C-reactive protein) and ESR (erythrocyte sedimentation rate) in the blood. If your ESR or CRP results are markedly elevated without an obvious cause, you need to have your healthcare provider investigate a little deeper. If your results are within the normal range, you can use your body's symptoms to help determine whether you are 'inflamed' or not.

You may have excess body inflammation if you have:

- heavy and excessively painful periods
- severe premenstrual symptoms including low mood, swollen hands, or sore breasts
- abdominal symptoms such as bloating, reflux, abdominal pain, or constipation
- unexplained weight gain especially around the midriff
- skin flushing or redness, feeling suddenly hot at times
- low energy and/or feeling unrefreshed and tired after sleep
- poor concentration with poor physical/mental stamina
- whole body aches and pains in the muscles, joints, or both
- irritability, unexplained anxiety, or low mood.

How to reduce whole-body inflammation:

- Optimize your gut health
- Reduce excess stress

Optimizing gut health

Optimizing your gut health is essential when striving to reduce inflammation and achieve better health. Your gut has an astonishing surface area of at least 30 square meters, and a substantial proportion of this interfaces with the bloodstream.[229]

This is why the gut-bloodstream barrier is so important and why 'gut permeability' (also called 'leaky gut') has become a hot topic of research.[230] If you have inflammatory molecules inside your gut, you can imagine that this could cause inflammation within your gut wall. This, in turn, could cause inflammation in your bloodstream and then in your whole body.[231] One of the most well studied groups of inflammatory molecules in the gut are *lipopolysaccharides* and these have been associated with inflammatory bowel bacteria and whole-body inflammation.[232] It turns out that having inflammatory molecules within your gut can increase the likelihood that your gut 'leaks' out these inflammatory molecules into the bloodstream. It makes sense, therefore, that you can help reduce your whole-body inflammation by reducing inflammation in your gut.

Reducing gut inflammation has a lot to do with improving your gut bacteria, or flora in the large bowel. In turn, this has a lot to do with what you eat and the health of your stomach and small bowel.[233] In other words, what you eat and how you digest directly influences what ends up feeding your *large bowel* gut flora, your all-important *microbiome*. How digestion in the mouth, stomach, and small bowel influences gut bacteria, and thus whole-body inflammation, has proven challenging to study.[234, 235] There are a number of ways in which the gut's digestive function can be interfered with, so before I cover how to remedy gut problems, I will start with a quick review of digestion and where it occurs.

Digestion of food starts in the mouth with chewing and saliva that contains fluid and enzymes. Food then passes down the esophagus, where it is transited rather than 'digested'. When it arrives in the stomach, food is mixed with acid and other secretions. Depending on the type and quantity of food, the stomach may take between 1.5 and 4 hours to signal to the gut that it has completed its task with the food. The food then passes through the small opening between the stomach and the first part of the small bowel. Here, a wider variety of digestive juices are poured out from the pancreas and gall bladder (bile) so that further breakdown of the food can occur in preparation for the main role of the rest of the small bowel, which is absorption of nutrients. Food stays in the small bowel for around 4-5 hours before it is moved into the large bowel, which as stated above is the part of the bowel that contains your gut flora or microbiome.

As you can appreciate, both the movement and digestion of food relies on various parts of the gut carrying out and completing their particular task, then signaling their activities to other parts of the gut. Correct signaling is paramount for the healthy movement and digestion of food within the gut. Without an optimal 'stomach phase' for example, you may reduce the efficacy of the 'signaling' for the next phases of digestion which involve digestive enzymes from the pancreas and gall bladder.

Symptoms of poor digestion, including heartburn and bloating
There are few medical tests that you can do to determine the health of your digestion, so it is worth knowing some of the symptoms that could result from poor digestion. If your digestion is not working optimally, you may feel uncomfortably 'full' or 'heavy' in the upper part of the abdomen for several hours after eating. You might also feel some acid reflux (heartburn) or pain in the upper area of the abdomen. Some people may suffer loose bowel motions as a result, others may suffer constipation. These issues could result from food intolerance, inadequate stomach acid, and poor movement of food through the gut. Although acid reflux is often successfully relieved with acid-blocking medication, these medications only stop the pain and discomfort of the reflux, not the reflux itself. In other words, they don't help the gut malfunction that is causing the reflux in the first place. In fact, acid-blockers could be interfering with overall digestive function. For example, reduced stomach acid may lead to incompletely digested proteins in the diet which in turn may contribute to gut irritation and inflammation,[234, 236] suboptimal gut flora and food allergies or intolerance.[237]

There are no readily available tests to measure stomach acid, with the Heidelberg pH test rarely done outside research studies. Heidelberg studies have revealed that excess stomach acid is not linked to reflux symptoms (Zollinger-Ellison syndrome), even though most doctors and gut specialists tell patients their reflux symptoms are due to 'excess acid'.[238] Instead, the studies reveal that reflux disease is linked to *low* gastric acid. Nevertheless, acid blocker medications (e.g., 'proton pump inhibitors') can be effective because although there isn't an *excess* of stomach acid, blocking stomach acid is often effective in relieving the reflux symptoms. Acid blockers are also important in treating disorders such as peptic ulcer disease, Barrett's disease, and hiatus hernia.

Tips for optimizing digestion

Stop, sit down, and relax: This allows the 'rest and digest' activities to activate in your 'parasympathetic' nervous system carried by your vagus nerve.

Focus on chewing and enjoying the meal: This encourages you to chew the food properly before swallowing, breaking the food down and mixing it with enzymes from the mouth. It also leads to more 'satiety' or 'satisfaction' feelings following meals.

Sip warm water with the meal: This allows the enzymes to work on the food immediately because the enzymes work best at body temperature and less so at colder temperatures. Adding crushed ginger or lemon to the warm water can also help the digestion process.

Leave 3-4 hours between meals: This allows the process of digestion to complete and increases the efficiency of digestion. It also allows the small bowel to carry out its cleaning/clearing activities properly. Snacks like a piece of fruit only need 30-45 minutes in the stomach, rice may need around 90 minutes, beans around 120 minutes and a large steak up to 4 hours. Surprisingly, a snack of nuts can take up to 3 hours because they are high in fat and protein.

Avoid fruit during and within three hours of meals with meat: A small amount of fruit is okay, but a large amount can cause the meal's proteins to putrefy and be less easily and completely digested.

Still have reflux and bloating after following the tips?

If you also have loose bowels and undigested food in the stool, your pancreas may not be working properly, and you should ask your healthcare provider about doing a *stool elastase-1* measurement. If you don't have these complaints, a stool elastase-1 measurement may still be helpful, because if it is borderline low, poor digestion could be your underlying problem and you may find supplementing meals with acid tablets, such as betaine hydrochloride (betaine HCl), and/or digestive enzymes, very helpful. Studies suggest that no more than 1,500 mg betaine HCl should be used to help acidify a protein meal however, starting doses of only 500 mg are advisable to gauge a response.[239] You will need a healthcare provider who is experienced in acid and enzyme supplementation to assist you.

Helpful tips if you have acid reflux:

- Check with your healthcare provider about any further investigations you may need.
- Don't use acid tablets if you have had a peptic ulcer in the past.
- Use acid tablets with care if you have 'methanogen overgrowth'.
- Use betaine HCl only with protein containing meals.
- Start with 500 mg, taking tablet(s) halfway into or at end of a protein meal.
- If you don't feel any heartburn with 500 mg, you can try 2 × 500 mg tablets for effect.
- If you don't feel any heartburn with 2 × 500 mg, you can try 3 × 500 mg tablets for effect.
- If acid tablets are working, you will feel less bloated and less reflux symptoms after protein meals.
- If the acid tablets are not working or cause heartburn symptoms, stop using them.
- Digestive enzymes can be used at any meal, use liberally to gain an effect and stop using if no relief from bloating or reflux symptoms.

Reduce or eliminate sugary foods to reduce inflammation
In my clinic, some of my sugar-addicted patients with heavy menstrual bleeding have had a reduction in their bleeding after stopping their consumption of sugars. This is likely due to reducing their whole-body inflammation.

One of the most important ways that avoiding sugar reduces inflammation is by reducing the amount of a hormone called insulin. Insulin is the main hormone that controls blood sugar levels. Sugary or even high starch foods cause a spike in blood sugar levels, which is followed by a spike in insulin. Both high glucose and high insulin are linked to an increase in inflammation, especially when the sugars/carbohydrates are consumed in high amounts on a regular basis.[240-242]

Persistently high insulin levels can also increase your risk of the metabolic syndrome and type-2 diabetes. Both of these conditions increase your risk of getting other chronic diseases and certain cancers like pancreatic, liver, endometrial and breast cancer.[243-246] Having high insulin also favors the development of abdominal or visceral fat (intra-abdominal fat around the organs) which is highly inflammatory to our bodies.[247] On this note, be very careful to avoid high fructose corn syrup additives. High fructose corn syrup can strongly trigger inflammation and a build-up of the inflammatory-type of visceral fat. [248] You can greatly reduce your risk of diabetes or help manage your diabetes if you avoid high fructose corn syrup, excess sugars in general and optimize your vitamin D level.[249] Many packaged foods in the USA including bread and crackers contain high fructose corn syrup, so make sure you read all food labels and definitely give anything containing it a miss.

Reducing or stopping dietary sugar can be tough for some people because they are both emotionally and physically dependent on it. You can usually tell if you are dependent on sugars. You may experience regular intense cravings for sugary foods, while feeling an inability to resist the craving. You may then overeat the sugary food to relieve the craving, which makes you feel somehow 'better inside' after consuming it, at least temporarily. If you know you have sugar cravings, go easy on yourself, get advice on the best way to reduce sugars, and avoid the 'guilts' about not being able to resist them. Once you can become free of sugar cravings, you can say 'no' to sugary foods more easily. This is when you will be able to tune in to the adverse effects that the sugar may be having on your body or brain function.

Eliminate gluten-containing grains to reduce inflammation

A plethora of scientific studies have found that gluten, a plant protein or lectin, can cause a 'leaky gut' and thus gut inflammation and whole-body inflammation.[250, 251] The most prominent researcher in this area, Professor Alessio Fasano, says:

> During the past decade, there have been a growing number of publications that suggest that loss of mucosal barrier function in the gut may adversely affect the trafficking of various inflammatory molecules, ultimately causing chronic inflammation, including autoimmunity, in genetically predisposed individuals.[252]

That's a bit of a mouthful but, basically, the loss of mucosal barrier function is what is known as 'leaky gut' and, as Fasano says, it can contribute to whole-body inflammation.[253] It is also linked to allergic disorders like asthma,[254] autoimmune conditions,[255] neurodegenerative or inflammatory conditions[256] and Alzheimer's disease.[153] A gluten-free eating plan in many women can also reduce bloating, reflux, abdominal pain, and constipation. For *all* women, however, it is about reducing whole-body inflammation and the related symptoms. As I said previously, there are no standardized tests to monitor 'inflammation' outside of the ESR and CRP, so monitoring your own digestion and inflammatory symptoms is your best guide as to how you respond to a gluten-free or low gluten diet.

Accessing gluten-free food in the past was challenging because of the lack of availability and expense. Nowadays, however, through popular demand in the western world at least, gluten-free grains (including organic varieties) are easier and cheaper to source and can make home cooking a healthful adventure. I have been recommending both gluten-grain-free and total grain-free eating in my practice for at least five years. The whole-body benefits, not to mention women's health benefits, have been so profound that I could not comfortably leave it out of my list of what I *highly* recommend for women. When excess weight is an issue for my patients, I recommend stopping grains altogether for a period of time. As well as reducing the exposure to gluten, this also helps reduce the overall carbohydrate content of their diet. Take note that for the purposes of reducing inflammation, the aim is a 'low-gluten' diet, rather than a strict gluten-free diet. For example, depending on the individual, I often recommend eliminating gluten-containing grains/breads, cookies, and beer. If you have celiac disease, *all* dietary gluten must be eliminated and a lot more attention to detail is needed.[257]

Drawbacks of a low-gluten diet

Although research in adolescents with celiac disease who are eating gluten-free diets has found that gluten-free eating in young celiac patients is linked to poor nutrition, metabolic syndrome, and heart disease, this doesn't mean the gluten-free diet *causes* these diseases.[258] In fact, a close look at this research suggests the increased risk of these chronic diseases most likely occurred because the young study subjects substituted their usual gluten-containing foods with gluten-free packaged foods high in sugar and inflammatory fats. The take-home message is that when swapping out gluten-containing grains, avoid all heavily marketed gluten-free packaged foods because they are often laden with unhealthy inflammatory fats, refined sugar, and food additives, all of which are harmful to your health in the long term.

Gluten-fortified grains and cereals contain abundant B-vitamins and fiber, so when eliminating these foods, add a good quality multi-B vitamin supplement or eat nutrient-dense foods like liver (e.g., liver pâté), heart, or kidney on a regular basis. Also include an abundance of root vegetables, whole foods, and a variety of 'pre-biotic fibers' like acacia gum, glucomannan, inulin FOS, green banana flour, globe artichoke, and burdock root. Consuming a wide variety of prebiotic fibers helps to feed and cultivate a wide variety of beneficial bacteria, which in turn will help reduce inflammation. A word of warning about consuming pre-biotic fibers: take extra care if you currently or have previously had persistent bloating or abdominal pain. In my experience, most people with IBS (irritable bowel syndrome) can eventually tolerate a wide variety of fibers if they are introduced slowly, even if they have to do so one fiber at a time.

Avoid exposure to glyphosate to reduce inflammation

Cutting out gluten grains can greatly reduce your dietary exposure to a pesticide called glyphosate, which in turn may reduce your inflammation. Many gluten-containing grains come from crops that are sprayed with this pesticide. Most of these sprayed crops are also genetically modified to increase the amount of gluten within the grain itself and to allow it to be resistant to the killing effect of glyphosate. These crops often include wheat, barley, rye, and triticale. Other non-gluten grain crops like soybeans, rye, lentils, buckwheat, and millet may also be heavily sprayed with glyphosate, with the usage varying by region and farmer. Spraying crops with glyphosate can increase the yield of crops by a whopping 100-200%!

So, what is the problem with glyphosate? According to prominent toxicology scientist, Stephanie Seneff, glyphosate alone, but especially in combination with gluten, can cause increased gut permeability ('leaky gut'). [259] This could be the most important reason why there has been a marked increase in the number of people complaining of gut and other health problems when consuming gluten-containing grains.[260-263] Other researchers have found adverse effects on gut flora and this has been linked to an increased risk of celiac disease, inflammatory bowel disease, irritable bowel syndrome and mental health disorders including anxiety and depression.[264] More recently, glyphosate has been found to cross the blood-brain barrier and to trigger inflammation within the brain.[265] Ph.D. scientist Anthony Samsel says:

> Glyphosate is not toxic in the conventional sense, but it destroys our biology at the cellular level one molecule at a time through disruption of proteins and signaling. Integration of the glyphosate within our bodies' structural proteins is the reason it can cause of an array of diseases, unleashing a cascade of ill health effects like a slow cumulative poison.[259]

If you feel inclined, you can reduce the amount of glyphosate and other potentially harmful chemicals in your diet by focusing on an organic diet. You can get information on how to choose cleaner foods by looking through the Environmental Working Group (EWG) website. The EWG has carried out an enormous amount of research to help us cut to the chase where prioritizing healthy shopping and eating is concerned. Look them up on <www.ewg.org>. I discuss harmful environmental chemicals or xeno-estrogens later in this section when covering the Estrogen Clearing Program.

Celiac disease and gluten-free eating

If you have bothersome gut symptoms such as bloating and abdominal pain, and/or if you have an autoimmune disease already, I recommend asking your health provider about whether you need to be tested for celiac disease before stop eating gluten-containing foods. When you stop eating gluten, tests for celiac disease are much less likely to turn up positive even if you have celiac disease. If celiac disease is not suspected, and you're looking to improve your general health, it is safe to stop eating gluten-containing grains (wheat, rye, barley, etc.). After stopping gluten, pay close attention to any changes that occur in your body including improvements in abdominal bloating, joint aches, back pain and even in your mood and clarity of thinking. Provided you avoid sugary and packaged food substitutes and increase your dietary fiber, you will likely enjoy some weight loss (if you need to lose weight) and an improvement in your wellbeing.

Vegetables and berries that can reduce inflammation

Consuming fresh vegetables, berries, and herbs helps to reduce inflammation, because they contain multiple beneficial plant chemicals that favor *less* rather than more inflammation in the body. As Harvard Women's Health Watch says:

> All green leafy vegetables, fresh fruits, and fresh seeds/nuts are full of vitamins, minerals and phytonutrients that help reduce inflammation and promote health. The top vegetables in this regard include brussel sprouts, broccoli, cabbage, bok choy and cauliflower.

They also mentioned some of the foods that increase whole-body inflammation, including refined carbohydrates and sugars, fried foods, processed meat, and margarine (that contain inflammatory fats like trans fats).

Vegetables contain plant proteins called lectins, and lectins can be both inflammatory and anti-inflammatory when consumed.[266] The more inflammatory lectins are found in pulses and nightshade vegetables including, lentils, beans, soybeans, peas, peanuts, chickpeas, eggplant, capsicum, tomato, and white potato. I recommend avoiding eating too many of these foods if you have inflammatory joint or autoimmune issues. You can reduce the number of lectins in these foods by using a pressure-cooker when eating them (this helps to inactivate the lectins).

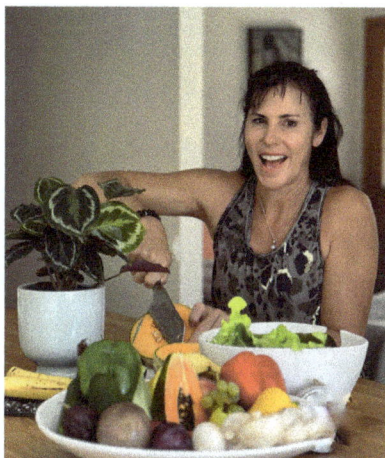

Tucking into some fresh fruit and vegetables

Dairy and inflammation

Cow's milk containing the milk protein called 'A1 casein' in some people can cause excess mucus production in the sinuses[267] and gut,[268] a problem that appears to be less likely with A2 milk.[269] A2 milk comes from Jersey cows and from the milk of goats, sheep, and camels. A1 milk differs from A2 milk in that histidine is in the place of proline in the milk protein. A1 β-casein milk is thought to slow the movement of food through the gut and to increase inflammation.[270] If inflammation or obesity is a problem for a patient, I recommend using A2 milk in preference to A1 milk and only in small amounts. I also encourage patients to try other milks that have a low carbohydrate, high protein and high calcium content, like coconut, cashew, macadamia or almond milk.

Oat milk is also a good source of calcium, but it tends to have a higher carbohydrate content than nut milk. Many women drink a large amount of dairy milk with their morning coffee and so rather than spoil the taste of the coffee with a nut or oat milk, I suggest they try substituting the milk with a small amount of pure grassfed cream or butter, both of which are very low in lactose and casein-protein. I found this to be largely well tolerated even by patients who report being dairy intolerant, and of course it is delicious!

Spices in your cooking can reduce inflammation

Spices contain thousands of plant compounds that help reduce inflammation directly (e.g., ginger and turmeric) or reduce inflammation via improving digestion. Spices can improve digestion by stimulating the liver to secrete bile that is rich in bile acids, components that are vital for fat digestion and absorption. They can also directly stimulate the activity of digestive enzymes.[271] Through their positive effect on digestion, various spices have also been shown to increase the absorption of important minerals like zinc and calcium, and they may even possibly reduce the risk of some cancers.[272] The most studied spices in this regard are ginger, piperine, cumin, capsaicin, curcumin, saffron, and garlic.

Animal proteins: Inflammatory vs. non-inflammatory

An animal protein may cause inflammation depending on:

- the type of animal
- how the animal has been fed and treated
- how the animal protein has been processed and packaged
- how you handle or digest the protein.

Surprisingly, chicken meat turns out not be healthier than red meat, and one of the reasons is that is has a higher proportion of omega-6 and other inflammatory fats than grass-fed red meat.[273] In fact, the proportion of the anti-inflammatory omega-3 fatty acids in grass-fed beef is greater than chicken, arguing against the commonly held belief that chicken is healthier than beef. Even so, it looks like chicken meat from hens that are grass-fed or are supplemented with flaxseed can achieve higher levels of omega-3 content and may be less inflammatory.[274, 275] It seems that what we feed animals may largely determine the degree to which eating their meat could be inflammatory. In the case of beef, the meat from animals raised in industrial feed lots is higher in saturated fat, contains unhealthy oxidized fats, has more inflammatory omega-6 fatty acids and contains toxic residues compared to free-range grass-fed animals.[276, 277] Unfortunately, given the structure of the meat industry and the logistics of mass production, if you are buying meat of any kind, such as beef, pork, chicken, duck, turkey, or lamb, unless the meat is labelled 'grass-fed', it comes from an industrially fed animal.

The other problems with consuming industrially raised animal protein relate to inflammatory toxic residues and the adverse effect on the environment. Feed-lot animals are fed predominantly grain, which is almost always sourced from grains that come from pesticide-sprayed crops. Moreover, compared to animals that are left to roam and freely eat grass, these animals are stressed, are more likely to be unwell and require antibiotics, and are more likely to be given hormones, all factors which can degrade the quality of the meat. If you consume red meat or chicken, I recommend visiting the places where the cattle or chickens are raised/fed, so you can get a true reality check about the conditions that industrially raised animals are subjected to. You may feel more motivated to eat less industrial meat and support local businesses

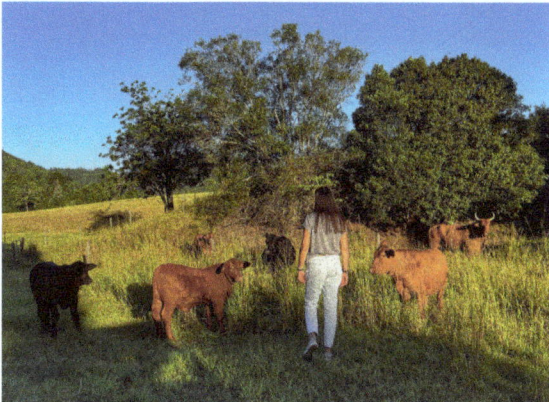

The beauty of regenerative farming: strolling through the herd

that use conscious, humane, and regenerative farming practices.[278] Regenerative farming incorporates rotational grazing, a technique that is critical to transforming over-used, over-grazed and eroded soils, to carbon-rich soils that can support future agriculture.[279]

In addition to choosing meat from non-industrial grass-fed sources, try to steer clear of processed meats. Processed meat is any meat that has undergone salting, curing, fermentation, smoking, or packaging with additives like preservatives. Studies suggest that consuming processed meats on a regular basis could cause a small increase in risk of cancer[280] and of dying of any cause.[281] While this sounds alarming, it is doubtful that eating small amounts of processed meats on occasion will be a problem.

Finally, once you have got your non-inflammatory pasture-raised fresh meat, don't spoil the health benefits by cooking it at extremely high temperatures in fats/oils. We all love barbecued meat, but when cooked in this way, your meat meal could be highly inflammatory, especially if you don't eat it with a mountain of leafy greens and other fresh vegetables like broccoli.[282, 283] Charred or barbecued meat contains a large number of inflammatory molecules called advance glycation end-products or AGEs.[284] These are what are responsible for the mouth-watering smell of barbecues, but when consumed on a regular basis, are inflammatory and could increase your risk of getting diabetes and heart disease. For a less inflammatory meal, slow-cook your meat in juices, and eat it with plenty of vegetables. For the occasional barbecue, lower your exposure to AGEs by eating it with a mountain of vegetables, a zinc capsule, and sipping warm water with lemon juice with the meal (extra acid for digestion).[285]

The chicken and the egg

As mentioned above, chicken meat may not be as healthy as previously thought. It is high in omega-6 fatty acids and if industrially raised, contains much of what chickens are fed including pesticides from pesticide-laden grains and animal by-products. Products called 'chicken meal' or 'chicken fat' are likely to have the highest concentration of inflammatory fats, inflammatory proteins, and chemical/pesticide residues, and these are common ingredients in fast foods and packaged food.[286] These products also often form the basis of pet food. Similarly, the composition of eggs reflects what the chickens are fed. Avoiding inflammatory components by choosing pasture-raised eggs can support your own health and the forward-thinking chicken farmers. Truly free-range chickens are better for the environment and the animals aren't subjected to cramped caged conditions. One egg contains 6-12 g protein, depending on its size. Most people can eat at least two eggs a day with no adverse health effects; in fact, most people who eat two eggs a day will experience a rise in their 'good cholesterol' called HDL (high density lipoprotein).[287]

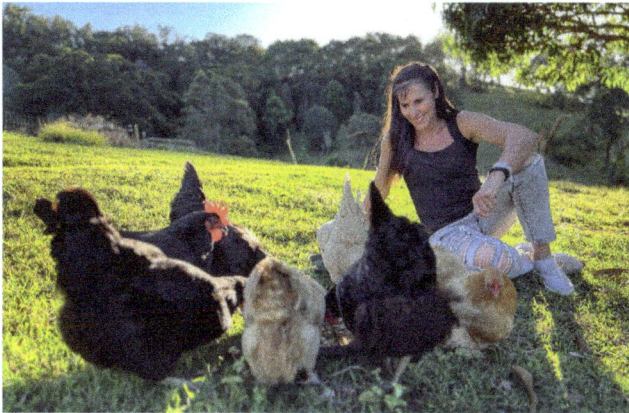

Greeting and feeding the chooks (Aussie slang for *chickens*)

Fresh, wild, small fish are the fish of the day

When you are looking for a seafood meal for your anti-inflammatory eating program, you want to avoid large varieties of fish including swordfish, flake (shark), orange roughie, marlin, Spanish mackerel, grouper, tilefish, farmed catfish, and tuna. These large varieties have fed off the food chain for several years, picking up pollutants, micro-plastics, dioxins, and heavy metals like mercury along the way. Instead, choose small non-farmed, wild-caught varieties like herring, mackerel, trout, tilapia, sardines, small wild salmon, anchovies, oysters, squid, clams, and mussels. These smaller varieties are cleaner and richer in anti-inflammatory omega-3 fatty acids, calcium, and other nutrients. Other reasonable choices include sole, flounder, cod, snapper, lobster, scallops, shrimp, and crab, but these are not as high in healthy omega-3s. When cooking fish, use low cooking temperatures with plenty of moisture to avoid producing inflammatory AGEs, and include fresh vegetables. If you like raw fish and sushi, you may need to make your own in order to avoid the large, farmed varieties and the kind of rice that is full of an array of chemical fillers. For healthy fish varieties, you can go to the Environmental Working Group website (<www.ewg.org>) and look up their summer seafood guide or join a community-supported fishery to find out what's what in fish; for example, <www.localcatch.org> in the USA.

Increase your protein intake at midlife and beyond

Protein requirements increase with age, which is somewhat counter-intuitive.[288] Consuming 1.0 to 1.3 g of protein per kg of your body weight daily, combined with regular resistance exercises, helps reduce age-related muscle mass loss. This amount of protein has been proven to be more effective in counteracting muscle loss than the previously recommended 0.8 g per kg body weight.[289] Given this increased protein requirement, it is especially important to make sure you're not increasing your consumption of inflammatory or processed meats and that you use cooking techniques that reduce rather than increase inflammation.

Sufficient protein as we age is needed to help counteract:

- **sarcopenia:** age-related muscle wasting (linked to chronic diseases)
- the **metabolic syndrome:** a condition linked to diabetes and chronic diseases
- increased **oxidative stress** age-related diseases
- the loss of our ability to absorb micro-nutrients.

Reducing stress: A necessary step in reducing inflammation

Stress can negatively impact many of your body processes including your mood, metabolism, inflammation, and immunity.[290, 291] It also seems to increase the likelihood of developing cancer and can make you age faster and look older.[292] Moreover, being excessively stressed can worsen or magnify any physical problems you have in a kind of unhealthy 'feed-forward' cycle. In this way, managing acute stress is as important as managing chronic stress, because both can be detrimental to physical and mental health.[293]

Many of the adverse effects of stress including inflammation appear to be mediated by the autonomic nervous system, the part of your nervous system that governs the automatic body processes like digesting, breathing, heart function, sexual function, etc.[292] Stress-reduction techniques can help reduce inflammation by deactivating the more inflammatory side of the autonomic nervous system called the sympathetic nervous system. I explained the sympathetic and parasympathetic nervous systems on **page 86** in **Section Two**. Most stress reduction techniques work by stimulating the parasympathetic nervous system which, in turn, helps reduce the activation of the sympathetic nervous system. The techniques are often called vagal stimulation techniques, because stimulating the vagus nerve increases parasympathetic activity (or 'tone'), and as a result produces widespread calming effects in the body.[294]

> **Mindfulness techniques that increase vagal tone include:**
>
> - mindfulness breathing, belly breathing, and alternate nasal breathing
> - heart rate variability training
> - yoga, qi gong, breathing-stretching
> - calming visualization, gratitude thinking
> - vagal stimulation through trans-auricular stimulation.

The most well-studied ways to deactivate stress pathways involve mindful breathing, and there are a handful of techniques. One well-studied de-stressing breathing technique is heart rate variability (HRV) training, a technique that relaxes the stress pathways and activates the rest/digest pathways in your body. I covered HRV training in more detail on **Section Two**. Other breathing techniques include alternate nasal breathing,[295, 296] diaphragmatic 'belly breathing',[297] and Zen breathing.[298] Yoga and qi gong[299] are ancient traditional techniques that act on specific non-physical or energetic pathways in the body and have widely published benefits.[300] Even simply stretching while deep breathing is more effective at improving heart rate variability than just doing either one.[301, 302] Another way to increase vagal tone is to 'greet the morning sun' (sun salutations) which also seems to help regulate your brain's circadian rhythm, and improve your sleep and metabolism.[303] Finally, gratitude journaling has been shown to vastly improve wellbeing, reduce anxiety and reduce resentment.[304]

De-stressing with color-breathing and stretching

I have devised an easy routine that combines some well-studied relaxation techniques including stretching, belly-breathing, and visualization. Many meditation techniques utilize imaginative visualization to make it easier to focus your mind and 'energy' into your physical body. The techniques are based on the concept that energy is *consciousness*, and that consciousness is *energy*. By using your imagination, you can direct your consciousness, or your body's energy to anywhere inside or outside your body. Research has shown that people can effectively use prayers or visualization of positive energies for healing and wellbeing purposes.[305] Even if you don't resonate with the existence of 'healing' energies, you can use visualization and breathing to bring yourself into the 'now' moment, where you are naturally more resilient to the stress-inducing chaotic conditions around you and within you.[306]

Visualizing moving colors often helps people become more aware of their energy or consciousness. In the morning routine presented here, you will be visualizing *swirls of pearlescent, silvery light*. Any combination of light pastel colors will do, so you can choose the combination of colors that you feel most comfortable with. Start with the color-breathing visualization technique while resting, then continue 'color-breathing' throughout your 10-minute stretch routine.

Color-breathing technique for your stretch routine:

1. Close your eyes and take some easy, deep, slow breaths.
2. Imagine yourself surrounded by silvery pastel colors that gently swirl around you and through you. Imagine these silvery pastel colors represent your body's energy or consciousness.
3. Each time you take a long inhale, imagine filling every single cell in your body with beautiful silvery pastel-colored light.
4. Each time you slowly exhale, intend to fully relax while feeling the nourishment that the in-breath delivered to the cells of your body.
5. Imagine this silvery pastel-colored light is *conscious*, and that you are filling your entire body with conscious healing energies.
6. While gently continuing with your color-breathing, move into the stretch routine.

The 20-step stretch routine

This routine involves getting on the floor with mats, cushions, or other support items to help you relax, focus, stretch and breathe. To fully relax during the stretches, set yourself up next to a bench, table, or chair that you can lean on. You may also want to have a cup of herbal tea or warm water beside you and a blanket or sheet to cover yourself at the end. In each position, take at least *three* long, slow color-breaths in and out remembering to bring your 'energy' or 'consciousness' into your body. Always be gentle with yourself and take more breaths in each position if you feel the need to.

A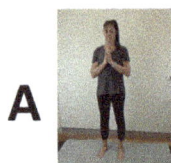

B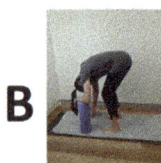

C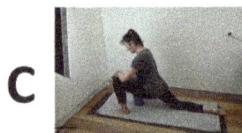

D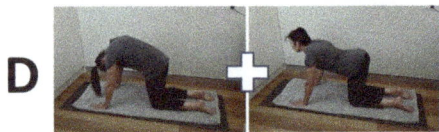

E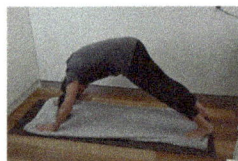

F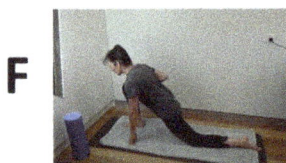

G 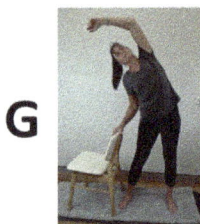 H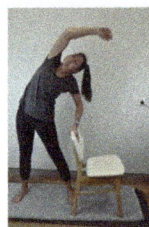

I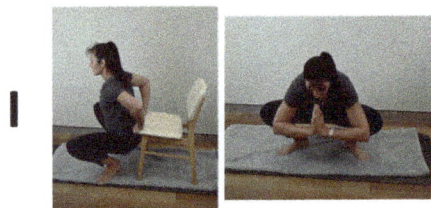

J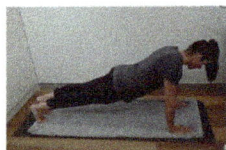

K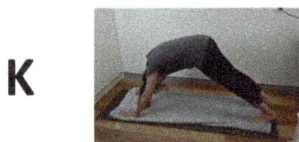

L 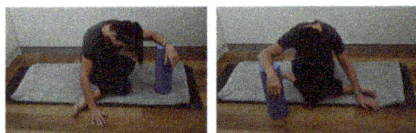 M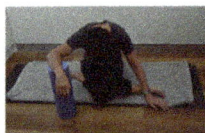

N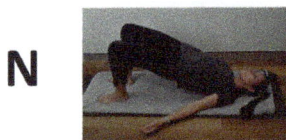

O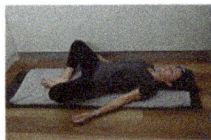

R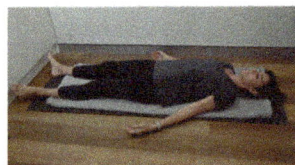

P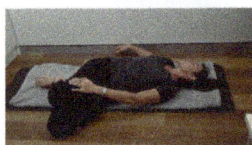

Q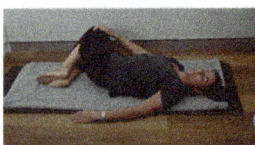

'R' for rest

1. **Figure A.** Stand with your hands in the prayer position in front of your heart with your legs together. Take at least **one** long, slow breath in and out.

2. **Figure B.** <u>Forward fold 1</u>: Inhale and reach your hands above your head, and using support if needed, slowly bend forward with your legs slightly bent, and exhale. While in this 'forward fold' position, take **three or more** long, slow breaths.

3. **Figure C.** <u>Forward left lunge</u>: Place your right foot behind you and place your right knee on the ground (left foot remains forward) and while feeling the stretch, take **three or more** long, slow breaths.

4. **Figure D.** <u>Four-point back stretch</u>: Bring your left foot back and place your left knee next to your right. Square yourself on all fours. Take **three or more** long, slow breaths while hollowing your back out towards the floor on the **inhale** and curling your back up in the opposite direction towards the ceiling on the **exhale**.

5. **Figure E.** <u>Down-dog 1</u>: Bring your buttocks up from all fours and position yourself in a down-dog position. Don't strain, and don't do it if it isn't comfortable. In this position take **three or more** long, slow breaths, feeling the stretch at the back of your legs. You can benefit from this even if you are pretty inflexible like me!

6. **Figure F.** <u>Forward right lunge</u>: Place your right foot forward, keeping/placing your left knee on the ground under you to support you. Feel the stretch while taking **three or more** long, slow breaths.

7. **Figure G.** <u>Standing sideways stretch to the right</u>: Using the support from a chair on your *right* side, while standing, bend at the hips sideways towards the chair while supporting your weight with the chair. When you bend as far as comfortable without bending forward or backward, add to the stretch by taking your left arm up and over your head. Take **three or more** long, slow breaths and feel the stretch in your left shoulder and whole left side.

8. **Figure H.** <u>Standing sideways stretch to the left</u>: Do the same as for step 7 but to the other side. Take **three or more** long, slow breaths and feel the stretch in your right shoulder and whole right side.

9. **Figure I.** <u>Squatting prayer 1</u>: This position is great for the hips, knees, and feet. Most of us have to start doing this by sitting on a pouf cushion or foot stool because of knee pain, stiffness in the hips, or pain/stiffness in the feet. It is worthwhile getting yourself into the position to some degree, because you will improve quickly. If desired, bring your hands together in front of you in the prayer position while taking **three or more** long, slow breaths.

10. **Figure B.** <u>Forward fold 2</u>: Refer to step 2 above.

11. **Figure J.** <u>Front Bridge</u>: This is for strength/resilience and can be skipped if you're not feeling up to it. Take **one or more** long, slow breaths here.

12. **Figure K.** <u>Down-dog 2</u>: Take **three or more** long, slow breaths here, feeling the stretch at the back of your legs.

13. **Figure I.** <u>Squatting prayer 2</u>: Refer to step 9.

14. **Figure L.** <u>Right-cross-leg forward bend</u>: Roll back onto your buttocks and cross your right leg over your left. If you can, cross your legs over further so your right knee sits on your left knee. This takes practice. Using the support of a chair or foot stool, lean forward and while taking **three or more** long, slow breaths, feel the stretch in your back, buttock, thighs, and elsewhere. Be gentle and don't overstretch.

15. **Figure M.** <u>Left-cross-leg forward bend</u>: Change position so that your *left* leg is now over your *right*. Using the support of a chair or foot stool, lean forward while taking **three or more** long, slow breaths.

16. **Figure N.** <u>Back bridge</u>: Lie back and bring your knees up and move your feet towards your buttock. Keep your hands facing down beside you. Using the muscles at the back of your thighs, raise your hips in the air as far as what is comfortable. Take **three or more** long, slow breaths while feeling a stretch in your back and thighs.

17. **Figure O.** <u>Hip stretch</u>: While relaxing on your back, bring the soles of your feet together and allow your knees to flop out to the sides. Take **three or more** long, slow breaths and feel the stretch in your hips and thighs.

18. **Figure P.** <u>Lying twist to the left</u>: Bring your knees together and have your feet flat and comfortably on the ground near your buttocks. Slowly let both your knees/legs fall to the *left* and let them fall as far as it is comfortable, if not all the way to the ground, while keeping your shoulders flat on the

ground. Prop your knees up off the ground if you need to in order to keep your shoulders flat on the ground. Take **three or more** long, slow breaths here while feeling the stretch in your back.

19. **Figure Q.** <u>Lying twist to the right</u>: Bring your knees and legs back to the center and this time, slowly let your knees/legs fall to the *right*. Let them fall as far as is comfortable, if not all the way to the ground, while keeping your shoulders flat on the ground. Prop your knees up off the ground if you need to. Take **three or more** long, slow breaths here while feeling the stretch in your back.

20. **Figure R.** <u>R is for rest and a time for *tuning in* to your body</u>: Bring your knees and legs back to the center and straighten your legs out. Let your legs and arms relax, with palms facing up. Cover yourself with a blanket or sheet if you wish, enjoy some long slow breaths, and take as long as you like. This position is an important space in time for *You*.

After your color-breath stretching, take the opportunity to contemplate:

- Am I really at peace regardless of the turmoil around me?
- What else should I be doing to take care of myself?
- What do I need to do to put my unique life purpose into action?
- How can I be more of service to others?
- How can I strengthen my family and community connections and wellbeing?
- Is there anything I have forgotten to be grateful for?

The Basic Program at-a-glance

To optimize gut health:

- Stop, sit down, and relax while eating.
- Focus on chewing and enjoying your food.
- Sip warm water with meals (+/- fresh lemon or ginger).
- Avoid icy cold drinks with meals.
- Tune into how your stomach feels during, and after meals.
- Avoid eating fruit within 2-3 hours of a high protein meal.
- Fast for 12-14 hours overnight.
  Consider getting advice on:
  – digestive enzyme support
  – acid support for protein-rich meals.

What an anti-inflammatory diet looks like:

- Reduce or eliminate sugary foods, candies, cakes, cookies.
- Reduce meals containing bread, rolls, toast, wraps or crackers.
- Favor nutritious meals with proteins, healthy fats and fiber.
- Eat any grains sparingly and use only organic versions.
- Eat 1-2 cups leafy greens and/or cooked vegetables every day.
- Include high-fiber root vegetables 2-3 times a week (pumpkin, swede).
- Consume milk sparingly and favor A2 varieties.
- Include high-calcium foods like seed, nuts, and greens.
- Favor organic versions of the Dirty Dozen™ vegetables and fruits (**page 144**).
- Use fresh herbs in salads and as garnish.
- Cook with spices (e.g., cumin, coriander) to help digestion.
- Pressure-cook pulses, beans, and nightshade vegetables (lectins).
- Eat only organic pasture-fed chicken eggs (or duck eggs).
- Eat only organic or pastured-fed chicken (max 2-3 meals a week).
- Choose grass-fed red meats or wild venison, kangaroo, or other game meats.
- Eat only locally caught small, wild varieties like sardines, herring, and mackerel.
- Avoid too many char-grilled or barbecued meat/chicken meals (increases advanced glycation end-products).
- Use moist low-heat cooking methods for meats, chicken and fish.

Fiber supplements:

- 10-15 g **soluble** fibers daily:

  Examples include guar/acacia gums, inulin FOS, GOS, green-banana flour, globe artichoke, apple pectin, glucomannan. Always start with small amounts ½ tsp (~2 g) and build up to 20-30 g depending on what you can tolerate.

- 10-15 g **insoluble** fibers daily:

  Examples include organic sprout powder, psyllium husks, seed mixtures (take care with these if you have any irritable bowel and bloating problems).

Reduce stress:

Get into a daily routine of breathing stretching and tuning into your body's consciousness/energy.

Give your body time to adjust:

Depending on your start-point, your body likely needs at least *three* months to adjust to the various components of the Basic Program. You know you have made progress when you become increasingly aware of the unpleasant effects of falling back into previous unhealthy habits. You may also be surprised how personally 'in tune' you are becoming and how much understanding you now have of the 'inflammatory' nature of some foods and lifestyle habits.

The Solutions

The Estrogen Clearing Program

The Estrogen Clearing Program

This Program is a diet and lifestyle program that assists your body in eliminating or clearing its own estrogen. Our ability to clear our own estrogen is not always optimal and its efficiency depends on our genetic make-up, our general health, and what we're exposed to in our environment and diet. You might be thinking that hormones like estrogen sort of 'fall out' of the body soon after they are produced when they are either not needed anymore or are in excess. Not quite. The body has a specific detoxification process involving packaging and transportation so they can be eliminated via the kidneys or bowel. This program is to help women process and clear their own and other estrogens because at midlife, women may have a higher load to handle, and in some, the elimination process may not be working optimally.

Why is an Estrogen Clearing program important for midlife women?

- A rise in estrogen may increase your risk of hormone-dependent cancers over time.
- Any hormone therapy that you may need after Zone 3 or Zone 4 could add to estrogen's cancer-causing effect over time.
- Environmental estrogens or xeno-estrogens add to the steroid hormone load that your body must process and expel.
- Few medical doctors appreciate the importance of Estrogen Clearing in your current and future health, so it is best to know how to take steps yourself.

Estrogen Clearing = estrogen breakdown and elimination = detoxification

Just as the production of hormones needs to be tightly regulated, so too, does the clearance of hormones from the body. Hormones are among the many molecules produced in the body that are eliminated via highly specialized processes. Your body constantly monitors the elimination of your hormones so it can promptly adjust the level according to its needs. Like most other hormones, estrogen is processed and eliminated by first *altering* the hormone, then *packaging* it with another molecule, then finally *transporting* it out of the body via the kidneys or bowel.

Alteration: Phase I

Estrogen is broken down into several different compounds called *estrogen metabolites*. This process takes place primarily in the liver but also in other parts of the body. This step is known as *phase I detoxification*.

Packaging: Phase II

Estrogen metabolites from *phase I* are made into packages that can be easily cleared from the body. This step is known as *phase II detoxification* and involves 'conjugation' or joining molecules to the phase I estrogen metabolites. This conjugation process forms phase II molecules that can be more easily eliminated from the body than the more toxic phase I molecules.

Transportation: Phase III

In phase III, the phase II conjugation compounds made in the liver are transported into the bile or directly into the bloodstream. The estrogen compounds that end up in the bile are passed out with the bile into the upper small intestine. From there, they are either reabsorbed into the bloodstream or passed out to the toilet. The phase II estrogen compounds that go directly into the bloodstream are eliminated from the body via the kidneys and urine. These steps are sometimes referred to as *phase III detoxification*. As you can imagine, you need to have plenty of water and healthy regular bowel movements for these steps to be successful.

When I first became a specialist medical doctor, I did not know about estrogen detoxification, let alone whether it was important or not. I did not come across it in my basic or specialist medical training and it was not on my radar when I was doing my women's health Ph.D. It was only after my Ph.D., when I was training in functional medicine, that I learnt about what it was and how it can impact our lives. Knowing the complexities of estrogen detoxification allowed me to appreciate that many of the symptoms that midlife women complain of could be explained by poor detoxification mechanisms. Although understanding the principles of estrogen and other hormone detoxification is not simple, the concepts form the basis of straightforward diet/lifestyle strategies that women can easily implement.

I don't know why we don't learn more about the body's hormone and other detoxification systems in our medical training, but it likely relates to the fact that there are no medications available to improve or speed up the process. Our primary focus in medical training is to 'right the wrongs' or give a 'pill for an ill', so to speak, and we don't learn about between-patient variations in detoxification and elimination. In fact, we don't learn about how variations in normal functioning in general can cause symptoms, because variations in *normal* function are not considered important because they are not a 'disease', are not serious, and therefore do not require attention or medicating.

Estrogen break-down molecules can be a problem

There are at least three different types of estrogen molecules in the human body including estrone (E1), estradiol (E2), and estriol (E3). When these estrogens undergo phase I detoxification, they undergo a process which produces numerous toxic phase I metabolites. These metabolites can cause damage to the body, so they are quickly processed into non-toxic metabolites via phase II conjugation. Phase II conjugation involves the addition of a neutral molecule to the phase I toxic metabolite, rendering it non-toxic and readily transported from the liver into the bile or urine. One well-known phase I estrogen metabolite called 4-hydroxyestradiol-quinone is known to cause damage to your DNA. Excessive exposure to this toxic metabolite can leave you at an increased risk of errors in DNA replication and repair, thereby increasing your risk of cancer, especially breast cancer and other hormone-dependent cancers.[307, 308] Moreover, these and other toxic metabolites can cause a buildup of toxic 'free radical' compounds in the body, and these, in turn, can inflame and damage your body.[309] This is why phase II detoxification is so important because it clears the body of these toxic phase I metabolites.

Figure 11: Estrogen detoxification and elimination at-a-glance

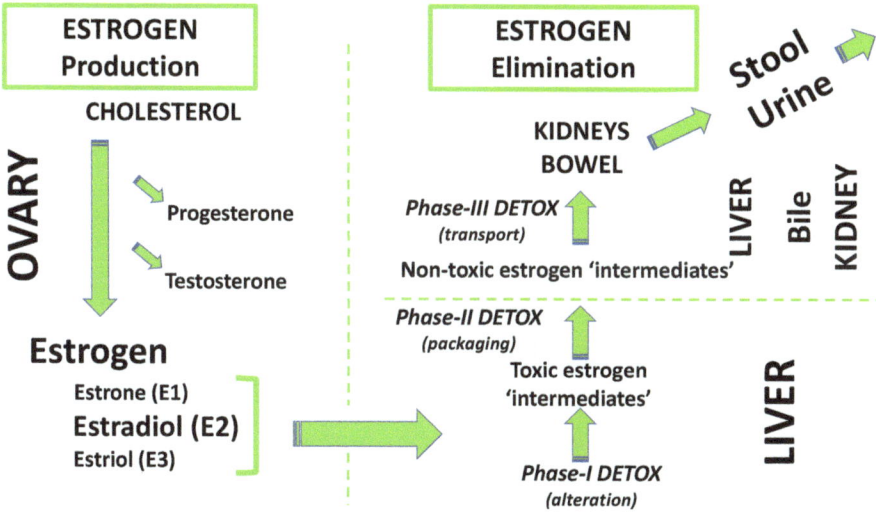

We are all different in terms of our body's ability to detoxify from estrogens and other hormones. Some of the differences are genetic, and these differences are known as single-nucleotide polymorphisms or SNPs. If we carry a genetic SNP that is linked to slow phase II detoxification, we are potentially more likely than others to run into issues with excess estrogen, particularly in our late 30s and 40s when estrogen levels can rise.[310] If we carry genetic SNPs that are linked to a fast phase I and slow phase II, we may find ourselves in even more trouble, because we may be exposed to a lot of phase I toxic metabolites that are not being cleared promptly in phase II.

There are also between-person variations in phase III detoxification. Remember phase III is where the non-toxic metabolites from phase II are transported out of the liver cells and eliminated from the body via the bile and bowel or via the bloodstream and kidneys. So far, the between-person variations in phase III detoxification are poorly understood, but in-lab and animal research suggest that both excess inflammation and excess estrogen may adversely affect it or slow it down significantly.[311, 312] This is why I emphasize reducing inflammation with the Basic Program as a necessary step before and during the Estrogen Clearing Program. The research in this area of body function is in its infancy, but in my clinical practice, I have observed women improve their estrogen clearance and related symptoms simply by reducing their whole-body inflammation.

Xeno-estrogens: Why women should know about them

The word *xeno-estrogen* literally means 'foreign estrogen' because 'xeno-' means 'foreign'. Xeno-estrogen is used to describe either naturally occurring or synthetic molecules that can interact with the body's receptors for estrogen. Both female and male bodies have estrogen receptors all over the body, and when estrogen circulates in the body, it can 'signal to' or give instructions to those parts of the body. Each part of the body will have a uniquely functioning estrogen receptor so that the estrogen signal can be specific to that part of the body. Like estrogen, xeno-estrogens can create signals within the body via their interaction with estrogen receptors. Naturally occurring xeno-estrogens are abundant in plants and therefore are often referred to as plant estrogens or 'phytoestrogens'. Phytoestrogens are especially abundant in soybeans, tofu, cashews, flaxseed, chickpeas, dried fruits, cruciferous vegetables, and legumes. Naturally occurring xeno-estrogens are also abundant in molds and fungi, and these xeno-estrogens are known as mycotoxins.

The effect that naturally occurring xeno-estrogens have on the body through their interaction with estrogen receptors is complex and although not always the rule, phytoestrogens tend to promote health, but mycotoxins tend to adversely affect it. Phytoestrogens have been studied in menopause because it was thought that taking phytoestrogens in food or a supplement could give the *benefits* of estrogen without its adverse effects. Before my Ph.D., I coordinated and published the results of studies on the effects of soy protein and red clover phytoestrogens on women.[313] We now know that phytoestrogens have some health benefits, but they don't have a strong enough estrogen effect on the body to significantly relieve menopausal symptoms or reduce the effect of aging on blood vessels.[314]

The most widespread and widely known synthetic xeno-estrogens are pesticides and plastics manufactured by the chemical industry. Because these have spilt over on a grand scale into the world around us, they are now known as *environmental pollutants* or *environmental toxins*. Examples that most people have heard of include bisphenol-A (BPA), and phthalates (see **Tables 8 & 9**), all of which interact with our estrogen receptors when inside the body. Because they interact so intimately with our bodies via the estrogen receptors, they are categorized as *endocrine disruptors*. Unfortunately, these endocrine disrupting xenoestrogens are everywhere in our daily lives including in most cosmetics, hair products, and plastics.

Pollutants as endocrine disruptors

Your own doctor is unlikely to tell you about environmental chemicals and their effect on our health because they, too, are largely uninformed about them unless they do their own research. Even those trained in Occupational Toxicology do not know much about environmental xeno-estrogens. One Australian toxicologist who took part in a research survey admitted the following:

> Hormone disrupting chemicals are not a consideration in our industry. We don't deal with the long-term problems. None of these molecular or unseen chemical injuries are being monitored. If you're talking about the millions of chemicals that are produced, gold standard studies are rare as hen's teeth on what these things actually do to people.[315]

We as doctors often assume that because we don't know about something in terms of health and disease, that that 'something' isn't important. Unfortunately, as a result, many doctors tell their patients that environmental chemicals are 'not important' or are 'fine'. But are they?

If you do your own research to answer this question, you will find a lot of information that is highly likely to alarm you. You can read a detailed account of xeno-estrogens and endocrine disruptors in an article by Claude Monnere, an article which is freely available to the public.[316] My own eyes were opened to the existence of xeno-estrogens and their widespread distribution when I was studying for my functional medicine certification. I learned that like all hormones, even in only tiny amounts, xeno-estrogens can have a dramatic effect on both animal and human health (especially child health).[317] This information is concerning when you come to understand it, especially given we are exposed to hundreds of them every day.[318]

When you do your own research, you may also discover that animals and humans will be heavily exposed to xeno-estrogens for decades to come with completely unknown consequences. In 2017, the U.S. chemical industry was worth more than $765 billion and has been increasing every year since. Since 1960, more than 85,000 different chemicals have been approved for use in commercial agriculture products, most of which have ended up in our food and water. As a result, hundreds of chemicals have been found in our bodies, including those of our unborn children. Only a handful of these chemicals have been tested in animals, let alone in humans, and none have been tested as combination cocktails.[319] A recent mini-review of BPA concluded that:

Many studies have shown that even very low exposure to BPA is associated with a range of chronic human health conditions, including diabetes, cardiovascular disorders, polycystic ovarian disease, hepatotoxicity, and various types of cancer.[320]

The United States Environmental Protection Agency (EPA) estimates that more than 500,000 tons of BPA leaches into the environment each year and over 90% of tested humans have detectable BPA in their systems with the highest levels found in infants and children. BPA is a common xeno-estrogen that remains in use in our food packaging and until recently was even used in baby bottles! As you will discover, the current and looming adverse health consequences are not getting the attention they deserve. As North American toxicologists Liza Gross and Linda Birnbaum at the National Institutes of Health say:

Existing U.S. regulations have not kept pace with scientific advances showing that widely used chemicals cause serious health problems at levels previously assumed to be safe. The most vulnerable population, our children, face the highest risks. More research is needed to better understand the risks posed by these chemicals, identify susceptible groups, and develop safe alternatives. But as the contributors (to this edition) also make clear, science is not always enough.[321]

The take-home message is that it is best to inform yourself about xeno-estrogens so that you can reduce your exposure to them. They are in many of the chemicals around us and that we ingest or absorb; they include persistent organophosphates (POPs), organochlorine pesticides, poly-chlorinated biphenyls, phthalates, and the widely used BPA. They are used in plastic bottles and food cans (BPA), medical devices (phthalates), detergents, flame retardants (polybrominated diphenyl ethers), toys (phthalates), cosmetics, pharmaceutical medications (parabens), and pesticides (alkyl phenols such as nonylphenol). This list will give you an idea of what the first step in the Estrogen Clearing Program entails, including avoiding pesticides, plastics, chemicals in foods, and chemicals in personal products, etc.

Why synthetic xeno-estrogens can be a problem
Both the amount of estrogen and the length of time we are exposed to estrogens contributes to the risk of getting hormone-dependent cancers like breast and endometrial cancer.[33] When I wrote a review about excessive estrogen exposure at midlife in 2002 with Professors Claude Hughes and Mark Cline, I was not aware that xeno-estrogens were also likely contributing to lifetime estrogen exposure. Professor Hughes, however, was aware. I remember he was already reading avidly about dioxins (polychlorinated biphenyls) and their adverse effect on the reproductive system! Since that time, the link between environmental estrogens or xeno-estrogens and cancer has been revealed and human studies have now confirmed a probable link between POPs and various cancers including breast cancer.[322]

It is not clear yet whether an excess of both estrogens *and* xeno-estrogens can cause symptoms in midlife women. As I have discussed, a rise in estrogen at midlife may be linked to heavy menstrual bleeding, breast tenderness, new-onset headaches, abdominal bloating, weight gain, irritability, and mood swings. Perhaps environmental xeno-estrogens could also be contributing? It is also possible that a combination of a rise in estrogen at midlife and xeno-estrogen exposure is important in increasing the risk of hormone-dependent cancers like breast and endometrial cancer. This possibility suggests that both women and doctors should be aware of environmental xeno-estrogens.

There are very few studies on the effects of xeno-estrogens in women, let alone midlife women. In one South American study, significantly more plastics and pesticide residues were found in the blood, abdominal connective tissue, and fat tissue of 120 obese women compared to normal weight controls.[323] The researchers also found that the amount of xeno-estrogens in the visceral and subcutaneous fat tissue was closely linked to impaired metabolism and increased markers of inflammation within the fat tissue. These findings lend weight to the argument that we need to address and improve detoxification when trying to lose weight. It is sobering to think that if environmental chemicals (including heavy metals) get stuck in our fat tissue, they probably also get stuck in our brains[324] which are comprised largely of fat and cholesterol. Once in the brain, one wonders how they can be removed before causing irreversible damage.[325, 326]

So far, there are no clinical studies to tell us whether eliminating excess estrogens and/or xeno-estrogens will reduce high estrogen-related symptoms or even reduce cancer risk. As far as heavy bleeding, breast tenderness, headaches, irritability, abdominal bloating, and weight gain are concerned, in my clinic, I have observed great improvements in women who have followed the combined Basic and Estrogen Clearing Programs.

Taking the steps to clear xeno-estrogens and estrogens

Clearing estrogens and xeno-estrogens from your body is about optimizing the three phases of detoxification in addition to maintaining healthy kidney and bowel function. All hormones and estrogen-like compounds in your body are eliminated through the complex detoxification system illustrated in **Figure 11**. Although no clinical study has been done to date to research what factors do and don't promote hormone and xeno-hormone elimination from the body, the suggestions outlined in the Estrogen Clearing Program come from some of the principles in animal and laboratory molecular research and what we know from nutritional science.

The steps in the Estrogen Clearing Program are easy to implement at home. They involve specific directions on diet and lifestyle and can be performed with or without supervision by a healthcare provider. While the Estrogen Clearing Program does not replace necessary interventions such as surgery, medication, or hormone therapy, it can reduce the need for, and increase the efficacy of, these interventions. Moreover, while all women should have a family doctor to keep tabs on their own and their family's health, positive diet/lifestyle interventions can reduce the number of doctor visits overall.

The Estrogen Clearing Program involves:

- Reducing your exposure to environmental xeno-estrogens.
- Improving detoxification through healthy kidney and bowel function.
- Reducing inflammation using the Basic Program.

Reducing your exposure to environmental xeno-estrogens

I believe an important part of the process of reducing your exposure to xeno-estrogens is to take interest in and become educated about the chemical world around you. This knowledge will hopefully give you the motivation to take affirmative action. There are a growing number of highly informative enthusiasts and experts on environmental toxicants who are contributing to a growing amount of information. Some of the most informative resources include the Environmental Working Group (<www.ewg. org>) and various books including *Healthy Home, Healthy Family* by Nicole Bijlsma, *The Toxin Solution* and *Clinical Environmental Medicine* by Joe Pizzorno and *Legally Poisoned* by Carl Cranor.

Tables 7 & 8 on pages 146 & 147 summarize some of the steps involved in avoiding xeno-estrogen-containing foods, personal products, beauty products, hair products, house-cleaning products, and plastics of all kinds. Swap out plastic containers for glass, use less plastic wrap, and don't heat/microwave any food in plastic containers (this increases the likelihood of plastics leaching into the food). Remember to read the label of anything that is sold as food in a packet. You may have to get used to putting them back on the supermarket shelf if there are a lot of chemicals on the ingredients list. Be particularly wary of the chemicals that have names ending in '-zol' or '-ene' or have a number in parentheses after the name. The chemical food industries are specialists at making packaged foods taste great, look appealing, feel nice in your mouth, resist clumping and to last a long time on the shop shelves.

Your choice of fruit and vegetables can also influence the load of xeno-estrogens that you and your family are exposed to. I inform my patients to look up the Environmental Working Group's Shopper's Guide to Pesticides in Produce for the Dirty Dozen™ and Clean Fifteen™. The Clean Fifteen are the fruits/vegetables that are the least likely to be heavily contaminated with pesticides so neither organic nor non-organic forms are likely to have a heavy pesticide content. The Dirty-Dozen are fruits/vegetables that are the most likely to be heavily contaminated with pesticides. So, when focusing on the Estrogen Clearing program, you should try to consume only organic produce whenever possible.

In 2024, the EWG's Clean Fifteen included avocados, sweetcorn, pineapple, onions, papaya, sweet peas (frozen), asparagus, honeydew melon, kiwi fruit, cabbage, mushrooms, mangoes, sweet potatoes, watermelon and carrots (eggplant, broccoli and cauliflower no longer make the list). The EWG's Dirty Dozen included strawberries, spinach, kale, grapes, peaches, pears, nectarines, apples, bell and hot peppers, cherries, blueberries and green beans (tomatoes and celery were previously on this list).

A note about the Environmental Working Group: the EWG are a non-profit, non-partisan organization based in the USA which is dedicated to providing information about toxicants in the environment with little to no government funding. Amazingly, their findings are often ignored by policymakers, the public, and the medical community. See <www.ewg.org>.

What foods to eat to optimize detoxification

Aim to include as many colored vegetables in the diet as possible, and as a general rule, have your meal consist of at least 2/3rd different colored vegetables and about 1/3rd meat or fish. Any of the brassica vegetables, like broccoli, cabbages, collards, cauliflower, bok choy, etc., are excellent in a detox diet but because they are difficult to digest when eaten raw, they should be eaten well cooked. Other excellent sources of micronutrients that support liver detoxification are liver, heart, and kidney sourced from grass-fed animals. These organ meats are rich in phosphatidylcholine, selenium, glycine, B-vitamins, and minerals that promote liver detoxification.

What do I do about dairy, tea and coffee to optimize detoxification?

Milk can contain a plenitude of pesticide and hormone residues, so I recommend only small amounts of pure A2 full-cream organic or bio-dynamic milk (e.g., small dashes in tea and coffee). I also ask women who have irritable bowel symptoms, are dairy intolerant or have problems with malabsorption to find alternative healthy high-calcium foods like sardines, wild salmon, sesame seeds, chia seeds, seeds in general, almonds, organic tofu and organic soy milk. You can also consider making your own highly nutritious kefir with organic coconut milk. It is an excellent source of beneficial gut flora and can assist gut and general immunity. When drinking smoothies or hot beverages, it is relatively easy to swap out dairy milk for other milks including coconut, almond, macadamia, oat, organic soy milk and 'combination' milks. Small amounts of cheese and butter are usually okay, even for those who are dairy intolerant.

For coffee drinkers, in general, I recommend no more than 1-2 strong cups per day, and I normally don't have them change this for detoxification programs unless they have major issues with fatigue. If you are a coffee drinker, be sure to drink your coffee before 11 am, because it can have a negative impact on your sleep without you being aware of it. Optimizing the quality and quantity of sleep as much as you can is an important strategy for general health and is critical in promoting healthy Estrogen Clearing.

Table 7: Tips for low-toxicant eating

Tips for low-toxicant EATING	Pesticides and pollutants involved
Organic versions of the EWG's Shopper's Guide Dirty Dozen	OCs, OPs
Grass-fed and lean animal products because animal fat can be extra-laden with chemicals	PAHs, OCs, OPs, dioxins, PCBs, PBDEs
Avoid burnt meats and oils or char grill or barbecue, and instead use methods that allow animal fats to drip away	PAHs, OCs, OPs, dioxins, PCBs, PBDEs
Favor organic/biodynamic dairy foods	Estrogens
Avoid farmed salmon, or large carnivorous fish, and instead choose seafood according to the Environmental Working Group's Good Seafood Guide	Mercury, PBDEs, PCBs
Use glass, ceramic, or stainless-steel containers for heating and storing foods if hot	Phthalates
Avoid plastic water bottles, plastic travel mugs and avoid washing plastic food or beverage containers under high heat	Phthalates
Avoid using vinyl cling wrap and only buy canned foods that are BPA-free and BPS-free	BPA
Avoid high-fructose, corn syrup and rice syrup	BHT, BHA, benzoate, sulphites
Avoid processed foods containing artificial colorings and sweeteners	

KEY: **OCs** = organic chlorinated compounds; **OPs** = organophosphate pesticides; **PAHs** = polycyclic aromatic hydrocarbon; **BHA** = butylated hydroxyanisole; **BHT** = butylated hydroxytoluene; **PBDE** = polybrominated diphenyl ethers (persistent); **PCBs** = polychlorinated biphenyls; **BPA** = bisphenol-A (persistent); **Phthalates** = esters of phthalic anhydride, used as plasticizers to increase flexibility, transparency, durability, and to soften polyvinyl chloride

Table 8: Tips for low-toxicant living

Tips for low-toxicant LIVING	Pesticides and pollutants involved
Avoid non-stick pots and avoid buying stain-resistant clothing, carpet or furniture	PCBs, aluminum
Avoid products made with particleboard or medium-density fiberboard	Formaldehyde, solvents
Avoid laying new carpets, and plan to replace old carpets with non-carpet flooring	PBDE flame retardants
Choose paints, glues, and sealants etc. that contain low or no volatile organic compounds (VOCs)	Volatile organic compounds and solvents
Cover or replace older foam furniture and consider removing old carpets and padding	PBDE flame retardants
Review all of your personal products especially deodorants and antiperspirants and see EWG's 'skin deep' information: you *do* absorb the chemicals you put on your skin!	Phthalates, dioxins, PCBs, PBDEs
Use air filters or ionizers in your bedroom and office and have a few plants (they can remove airborne toxins)	Dust particles that trigger allergies, mold mycotoxins
Avoid living or working in mold-affected water damaged buildings	
Read more in the book 'Healthy Home, Healthy Family' by Nicole Bijlsma Ph.D.	

KEY: OCs = organic chlorinated compounds; **OPs** = organophosphate pesticides; **PAHs** = polycyclic aromatic hydrocarbon; **BHA** = butylated hydroxyanisole; **BHT** = butylated hydroxytoluene; **PBDE** = polybrominated diphenyl ethers (persistent); **PCBs** = polychlorinated biphenyls; **BPA** = bisphenol-A (persistent); **Phthalates** = esters of phthalic anhydride, used as plasticizers to increase flexibility, transparency, durability, and to soften polyvinyl chloride

Promoting healthy bowel function and bowel flora (microbiome)

A detoxification program can be perfect, but if your bowels are not working and/or you are not drinking enough pure water, all your efforts could be in vain. This is why I teach my patients to 'start at the bottom' first. Healthy detoxification and elimination via the bowel depend on opening your bowels regularly and easily and also a healthy, diverse large bowel flora or microbiome.

I will explain the importance of having an optimally functioning bowel this way. If you start to encourage phase I or II detoxification *before* your bowels are functioning optimally, you could find yourself feeling very unwell with both physical and mental fatigue. These symptoms are likely due to an abnormal buildup of both phase I and phase II metabolites within the liver and body. In other words, if these metabolites cannot be eliminated out to the toilet, they could effectively clog up the liver and other body parts. Although there has been no research into symptoms and related effects of poor elimination, in my clinical experience, it can be a major problem and I see toxicity symptoms in many of my patients with poor gut health and/or severe constipation.

Having poor bowel function and a suboptimal microbiome may also disrupt the normal circulation of bile between the gut and the liver, a process called the *entero-hepatic circulation*.[327] I discuss this process on **page 149**, and how it may lead to disrupted estrogen metabolism and excess estrogen problems.[328]

As previously mentioned in the Basic Program, one of the easiest ways to ensure optimal gut function is to supplement your diet with *soluble* and *insoluble fibers*. Fibers are forms of plant carbohydrates that are not digestible by the human gut. Because our gut can't break these fibers down into nutrients, they pass through the stomach and small intestine and into the large bowel, where they provide nutrition to our microbiome. The wider the variety of fibers we can consume, the wider the variety of beneficial bacteria that can be supported. The more beneficial bacteria making up your microbiome the better your estrogen clearing and detoxification mechanisms can function. Please refer back to **page 134** in the Basic Program.

If you have any degree of constipation, be careful with some of the 'gum' soluble fiber supplements, because in some people, they can worsen constipation. In fact, they are a good choice if you have the opposite problem and are looking to 'firm up' your loose bowel motions. In general, it is a good rule of thumb to experiment with small amounts of a few different types of fibers to find which ones suit you personally and aim to regularly consume a variety rather than only one or two of them. If you have a history of constipation, having a daily bowel motion may not be an accurate indicator of healthy bowel function, so have your doctor periodically check your progress with a simple abdominal X-ray. Regardless of what your healthcare provider advises for constipation, don't accept that constipation is either 'normal' or insurmountable. It will be worth every effort to find long-term healthy fiber solutions.

If you tend to have loose bowels, you may also need to be careful when introducing some of the fibers. Your gut may become 'irritated' by them initially, and you may get some cramping, excessive flatulence, and increased bowel movements. If this is the case, reduce the amount and frequency of the fibers, take one fiber at a time, then gradually increase them again. If you have a history of bloating and irritable bowel problems, prebiotic fibers can initially worsen your symptoms, but if you slowly increase them, over time, they will lead to improvements. It is a matter of trial and error and finding which fibers suit you best. As alluded to already, and although it isn't a hard and fast rule, I find the 'gum' and 'pectin' fibers tend to firm up loose bowels and the harsher insoluble fibers (psyllium husks) tend to make them looser. I encourage my patients to experiment so they can eventually take their own unique combination of fibers on a regular basis.

The role of your entero-hepatic circulation in detoxification

As mentioned previously the entero-hepatic circulation involves the circulation of bile acids in the bile between the gut ('entero') and the liver ('hepatic'). Only around 5% of the bile acids produced in the bile are eliminated with the bowel motion. Most of them are reabsorbed by the last part of the small intestine called the *ileum* and sent back to the liver for recycling into the next lot of bile. This recycling process means that the body only needs to produce about 5% of the total amount of bile that is circulating in the gut every day. As a consequence of this bile acid recycling, other compounds including phase II metabolites are also reabsorbed.[329] Little is known about what determines how many phase II compounds are eliminated vs. reabsorbed, but it may have something to do with the kind of microbiome you have.[330-332] Certain bacteria produce an enzyme called *beta-glucuronidase* and this enzyme can 'un-package' the phase II compounds, possibly leading to them being reabsorbed, but this is unlikely to be the only mechanism.[329]

Research suggests that a diet rich in fruits and vegetables such as apples, brussel sprouts, broccoli, and cabbage is linked to lower beta-glucuronidase in the gut.[333] These foods likely promote a healthy gut microbiome, which may lower the amount of beta-glucuronidase produced and in turn, lower the amount of phase II metabolites being reabsorbed.[334] Thankfully, research into the workings of the microbiome, estrogen metabolism and estrogen excretion continues to grow.[330, 331, 335] Calcium-D-glucarate is a supplement that has sometimes been used to promote the elimination of phase-II compounds by counteracting the actions of beta-glucuronidase. However, frequent high doses (at least 5 g daily taken in divided doses throughout the day) are needed to be effective.[336] Sometimes I recommend this supplement in women with high estrogen and xeno-estrogen exposure, but taking such high doses throughout the day can be too life-consuming to do on a regular basis or for long periods.

Promoting detoxification via the gut using 'binders'

Charcoal, bentonite clay, and apple pectin are compounds known as binders, because they 'bind' compounds in the gut and carry them out to the toilet. Binders play a role in reducing the reabsorption of phase II metabolites via the entero-hepatic circulation.[337] Oral activated charcoal has been shown to help mop up toxic or inflammatory compounds including lipopolysaccharides.[338] Avoid taking binders 1-2 hours either side of eating a meal, medications or supplements and they are not advisable at all if you are taking slow-release or controlled-release medications. Very few clinical studies have been done on the health benefit of binders,[337-340] so it is very much up to the individual and an experienced healthcare provider to work out a plan for you. I prescribe binders in my practice to help women detoxify if they have been seriously affected by a known environmental toxicant such as mold mycotoxins. I have women take 1-2 tsp activated charcoal with or without ½ tsp bentonite clay 5-6 days a week. I sometimes use higher doses of charcoal in women who have specific goals and tolerate it well.

Promote healthy bile flow with digestive bitters

Information about the role that bile and bile flow plays in promoting healthy digestion and detoxification was challenging to find in my medical and specialist training, and it was only briefly covered in my functional medicine training. So, I had little knowledge on the role of bile and bile flow in the detoxification pathway and considered it only important in the proper digestion of dietary fats. It is likely, however, that bile plays a critical role in maintaining healthy gut motility, gut hygiene (through its anti-microbial action), in addition to having a role in detoxification.[341]

As I explained in **Section Two**, bile formation and the gall bladder can malfunction in midlife women and many end up having to have their gall bladder removed. Bile and gall bladder problems seem to be common in women who have issues with bloating, gut motility (forward motion muscle coordination in the gut), excess estrogen and other symptoms of poor toxin elimination.[342] As I said in **Section Two**, I suspect that excess midriff weight in women with gall bladder issues relates to poor elimination and excess inflammation.[332] In **Section Two** I also explained that high estrogen can interfere with one of the phase III transport molecules. So, in some women, their own estrogen can be a kind of 'anti-cholagogue'. A cholagogue is a substance that encourages bile flow, so an anti-cholagogue would inhibit bile flow. Cholagogues stimulate both phase III in the liver and bile flow from the gall bladder into the gut. The cholagogues do this by binding to specific receptors called bitter receptors (T2R receptors). You may have heard about the bitter receptors on your tongue. It might surprise you, however, that we have bitter receptors throughout the entire digestive tract and elsewhere such as the lungs, kidneys, and the endocrine system.

'Bitter herbs' are those herbs that interact with the bitter receptors in the body.[343] They include but are not limited to dandelion, gentian, Oregon grape, and solidago (golden seal). Many other plant compounds are known to stimulate bitter receptors and have been used in Chinese and other traditional medicine as 'bitters' for centuries.[344] Similarly, traditional 'Swedish bitters' have been used throughout history in many European countries as pre-meal aperitifs to stimulate the digestion and bile flow and help guard against pathogens in the gut. The bitters in the lemon, lime, and bitters drink are also made of bitter herbs, including Angostura Aromatic Bitters®, a concentrated liquid made of gentian, herbs, and other spices dissolved in alcohol (the original recipe being from Trinidad and Tobago). This liquid is said to help cleanse the palate and facilitate digestion. I think, however, that most of us drink it for the taste, as it is a lovely refreshing summer drink with ice.

Digestive bitters for your kitchen table

As part of the Estrogen Clearing Program, I recommend combinations of bitter herbs including dandelion root, gentian, solidago (goldenseal), Oregon grape, myrrh, and wormwood in either alcohol or glycerine. You can purchase digestive bitters as a concoction or have them made up by a reliable herbalist. When you research bitters online, you will find several outlets that sell digestive bitters and other traditional Swedish bitters. You should start by taking only a few drops of the concentrated concoction in 200-300 mL (6.5-10 fl.oz.) of warm water at the start of your meal. If you are one of those people that cannot tolerate herbs and tinctures, you may need to keep it at a low dose, otherwise a usual dose would be a dropper full in 200-300 mL warm water. If you find you get loose bowels or are a bit more flatulent with the bitters, reduce the number of drops in accordance with your symptoms.

I have found bitters to be a game changer in women with excess midriff weight, bloating, and other complaints linked to excess estrogen and inflammation. If bitters are not your style, or you want some variety with meals, you can also use crushed ginger in warm water, taken with a meal. While ginger isn't a specific bitter receptor stimulator, it is excellent for the digestion,[345, 346] the microbiome[345] and general health.[347]

Ensuring healthy kidneys

Be sure to drink at least 1.5 L pure filtered water daily, *in addition to* any coffee or tea. 600-800 mL (20-27 fl.oz.) of this can be drunk as warm water when you get up in the mornings. One of the first things I do in the mornings is drink 300 mL of warm water with my prebiotic fibers and supplements. I then make a cup of hot herbal tea, which I sip slowly during my 20-stretch and color-breathing routine (**pages 125-129**).

Optimizing phase I and phase II: What to eat

The phase I and phase II detoxification processes occur in many parts of the body, but mostly in the liver. This is why phase I and phase II detoxification is also referred to as *liver detoxification*. As outlined in the Basic Program, the most important steps in promoting liver detoxification are to avoid pollutant-laden foods, inflammatory foods, excess alcohol, and the use of liver-damaging medications wherever possible (e.g., paracetamol and acetaminophen). If you are struggling with your symptoms or have stubborn excess weight, I recommend stopping alcohol for at least eight weeks then, if desired, resume a standard drink once or twice a week or on special occasions.

Foods that support detoxification:

- Watercress: [348] 1.5 cups daily improves phase II detoxification and protects from harmful products of phase I.
- Garlic:[349] 600-1200 mg twice a day (or 2-3 crushed cloves daily) stimulates phase II and up-regulates the body's primary antioxidant system.
- Beetroot:[350, 351] enhances phase II and protects from harmful products of phase I.
- Broccoli:[352] 'glucosinolates' in broccoli and other brassicas stimulate phase II and clearance of toxic phase I quinone metabolites.
- Berries:[353] including blueberries (contain proanthocyanidins) and stimulate phase II detoxification. Proanthocyanidin-rich foods also include apples, cinnamon, green tea, cocoa, pine bark extract and grape seed extract.[354]

Making your own 'detox shot'
Consuming detoxification-promoting foods on a regular basis can be exhausting to say the least! To make it easier, I suggest creating a supply of frozen

'detox-shots' that you can defrost and consume on a regular basis. Start by purchasing as many of the ingredients from the list below. Then, rather than storing them, while fresh, blend them thoroughly in a food processor. Divide the blended mixture into half-egg-cup-sized portions and freeze them in a manner that makes it easy to remove from the freezer when desired. When you are ready to use your single detox-shot take it out of the freezer and let it thaw before swallowing it quickly (like a 'shot'). Alternatively, you could add it to your favorite super-food smoothie.

Food extracts that support detoxification:

- Green tea extracts:[355, 356] contain 30% 'catechins' compared to black tea that has 4%. Reduces overactive toxin-producing phase I enzymes and promotes phase II including clearance of toxic quinone estrogens and is linked to a lower risk of breast cancer in Chinese women.
- Pomegranate extract:[357] 500-2,000 mg (contain ellagitannins and anthocyanins).
- Sulforaphane (broccoli extract):[358, 359] 30-60 mg.
- Artichoke:[360] 3-6 g (multiple health benefits including liver detoxification).
- Olive oil:[361, 362] 1-4 tbsp (contains hydroxytyrosol).
- Curcumin:[363] 600-2,000 mg.
- Quercetin: 500-2,000 mg.
- Spirulina:[364] 500 mg.
- Aloe vera juice:[365] 60-120 mL.
- Milk thistle:[366-369] 400-900 mg daily via capsule in divided doses. Safety profile well known, promotes phase II detoxification, protects from toxic phase I metabolites, and helps liver problems including disorders that tend to block bile flow.

The Super-Food Detox Smoothie

I have listed some ingredients below which you can use to make your own 'detox-promoting' shot or smoothie. Some people find drinking all these ingredients together is not a problem, while others need to add one ingredient at a time and take only small amounts. For the smoothie base, I suggest using 200-300 mL (6.5-10 fl.oz.) coconut water, cold hibiscus tea, almond milk, or organic soy milk. Aim to include 20-30 g protein from a clean source like organic hemp protein or grass-fed collagen protein and about between a teaspoon and a tablespoon of a supplemental fiber that you know you can tolerate. If you don't find the consistency or taste of your smoothie appealing, it may help to drink it icy-cold or add a dash of vanilla, cinnamon or honey.

Ingredient ideas for your Detox Shot:

- watercress (0.5-1 handful) or watercress powder (1-2 tsp)
- green tea powder (1-2 tsp)
- turmeric root (0.5 tsp crushed)
- spirulina powder (1-2 tsp)
- aloe vera juice (60-120 mL)
- organic broccoli sprouts or alfalfa (1-2 tbsp)
- beetroot (0.25-0.5 medium bulb)
- blueberries and/or blackberries (1 cup) or organic berry powders (1 tsp)
- barley grass powder (0.5-1 tsp)
- pomegranate seeds or unsweetened syrup
- parsley (0.25-0.5 cup) or cilantro (0.25-0.5 cup)
- fresh mint (1-2 leaves).

Ingredient ideas for your Detox Smoothie:

- organic celery (0.5-2 sticks)
- chia seeds soaked overnight (0.5-1 tbsp)
- organic apple unpeeled (0.5-1)
- avocado (0.25-0.5)
- fresh lemon or lime juice (1-2 tsp)
- globe artichoke (0.5-1)
- organic spinach or kale (avoid if sensitive to high oxalates)
- organic soaked oats (1 tbsp)
- sunflower seeds (0.5-1 tbsp)
- organic cocoa powder (0.5-1 tsp).

Vitamins, minerals, and other micronutrient supplements that promote liver detoxification

Many of the micronutrients that are important in liver detoxification can be acquired from a diet plentiful in fresh food. However, even fresh foods are not always nutrient-rich, and our busy lifestyles may mean we don't get the optimal amounts through diet.

I offer supplements to assist in detoxification when a patient is:

- slower than expected to respond to the Basic and Estrogen Clearing Programs after 1-2 months
- particularly unwell with their symptoms
- unable to access and consume a nutritious diet
- having problems with gut health that could be reducing nutrient absorption.

Below is a less-than-exhaustive list of commonly used micro-nutrient supplements that support the liver detoxification process. Because the detoxification process isn't widely recognized as important to human health, there are almost no clinical data on the kinds of supplements that help or might help. Most of the supplements that are recommended by naturopaths and other health professionals are those that have been found in laboratory experiments to be part of the chemical reactions involved in phase I and phase II chemical reactions in the liver, and other parts of the body. Many of these supplements below can be found in combination products sold as 'detox' supplements. In my experience, some of these can be helpful, so, despite the lack of clinical studies for many of them, I will often trial them for about three months. The supplements I find most useful are magnesium (this is a keeper for women's health in the long term), zinc, vitamin C, vitamin D, glycine and taurine.

One very important mineral that can become depleted at times of emotional and physical stress is magnesium. The most reliable forms of magnesium include magnesium citrate, glycinate, orotate, or chelate. If you take magnesium in divided doses through the day or in a slow-release capsule, your body can utilize the full dose more efficiently. If you take your magnesium in large amounts all at once, your kidneys are likely to remove a large proportion of the dose within an hour or so of ingestion.

Supportive micronutrient supplements for liver detoxification:

- magnesium citrate, chelate or orotate: 500-1,000 mg divided doses
- alpha lipoic acid:[370] 50-200 mg
- resveratrol:[371] 300-600 mg
- vitamin B12: 1,000-2,000 IU
- choline: 400-600 mg
- taurine: 400-600 mg
- vitamin B2: 30-60 mg
- vitamin B6 (P5P): 20-30 mg
- vitamin C: 2-4 g
- vitamin E: 2,000 IU
- selenium: 400 µg
- glycine: 750-1500 mg
- taurine: 500-1500 mg
- methionine: 150 mg
- zinc: 30-60 mg in form of citrate or bisglycinate
- molybdenum trioxide: 150 µg (depletes with heavy pesticide exposure)

What about supplements that work on phase I detoxification?

As I mentioned above, I do not recommend focusing on phase I detoxification through supplementation. The phase I enzymes and pathways are vast in number and are influenced by multiple factors.

The only specific phase I supplement I have used in the past is di-indoyl-methane or DIIM, which is derived from a brassica vegetable-derived compound called indole-3-carbinol. DIIM stimulates the phase I enzyme called CYP1A1, which favors the formation of less toxic phase I estrogen intermediates.[372] DIIM has been shown to have possible beneficial effects in breast cancer and breast cancer prevention.[373] Having said that, the only time

I use DIIM in my practice is if there are clear indications of estrogen clearance problems (determined on dried urine testing), after addressing all the aspects of phase II and phase III detoxification (discussed so far).

Table 9: The four principles of estrogen detoxification at-a-glance

1. Promote healthy bowel function and flora	How-Why
Abdominal X-ray to identify constipation if present and monitor regularly	Treating constipation is paramount in maintaining a healthy phase III detoxification process.
Eat a wide variety of vegetables *and* at least 15-20 g combined soluble and insoluble fiber supplement	Encourages healthy bowel movements and sustains a wide variety of healthy gut flora
Look into binders, including charcoal, and bentonite clay	Promote phase III elimination, reduce the reabsorption of phase II compounds
Follow the guidelines for healthy digestion in the Basic Program	Promotes healthy gut function, combats gut inflammation and assists phase III elimination
2. Encourage healthy kidney function	**How-Why**
Drink at least 1.5 L pure filtered water daily	Helps the kidneys 'flush' the phase II compounds into the urine
Avoid excessive acetaminophen, ibuprofen, naproxen, paracetamol, aspirin and other potentially kidney-harmful analgesic medication	Reduces the toxic load on your liver and kidneys
3. Promote healthy bile flow	**How-Why**
'Bitter' herbs (e.g., dandelion root, gentian, solidago)	Stimulates 'bitter receptors' in gut and liver to optimize bile flow, phase II & phase III elimination
Warm water and lemon (or vinegar) with meals	Encourages optimal digestion in stomach to send the correct 'messages' that optimize bile flow and pancreas function
Reduce alcohol to 1-2 standard drink three times a week or less	Increases the available detoxification pathways in the liver
Reduce inflammation using the Basic Program	For optimal phase II & III detoxification

4. Optimize phase I and phase II detoxification in the liver	How-Why
Reduce alcohol: if an alcohol enthusiast, limit to 2-3 glasses of wine no more 2-3 times a week.	Reduces the phase I metabolite load so both phase II & III elimination can be optimized
Reduce the use of liver-toxic medications like acetaminophen and paracetamol	Reduces the phase I metabolite load so both phase II & III elimination can be optimized
Include superfoods in your menu plan on a regular basis	Promotes phase II detoxification while balancing phase I
Include amino acids taurine, glycine, choline, methionine	Vital nutrients to help optimize phase II detoxification
Consider including other nutrients inositol, Co-enzyme Q10, zinc, copper, selenium, manganese, magnesium, vitamins A, C, E etc.	Support phase II detoxification
Consider including detox herbs like silymarin (milk thistle)	Support phase II and balances phase I detoxification

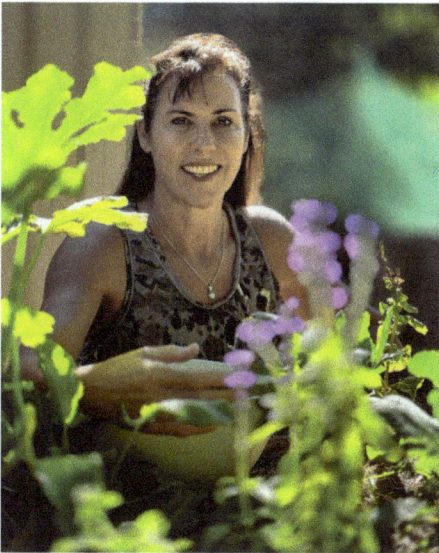

Harvesting our vegetables and herbs and getting out in the sunshine

Frequently asked questions about estrogen clearing

Will fasting help me succeed on the Estrogen Clearing Program?

We don't know for sure, but there are some indicators that it may be beneficial. One of the most popular fasting regimens is the 'fasting-mimicking diet, or 'time restricted eating'.[374] by Dr. Valter Longo at the University of Southern California. Dr. Longo says that intermittent fasting can activate specific inflammatory and immune responses that can accelerate the regeneration and repair of many parts of the body.[375] All these features would likely benefit the detoxification pathways in the body. Moreover, intermittent fasting seems to be as effective as calorie restriction diets for weight loss,[376] and it seems to have significant positive effects on diseases like diabetes,[377] obesity,[378] and autoimmune disease.[379]

What should I do if I have irritable bowel syndrome (IBS)?

If you have IBS, you probably experience regular bouts of bloating, abdominal pain or discomfort, constipation, loose bowels, or excessive flatulence. It is important to treat your IBS before or at least during any detoxification program, because if your gut is not working optimally, it won't be as efficient in terms of being able to help clear your estrogens and other toxicants via the stool. Tending to your diet, optimizing your digestion, and having regular bowel movements are paramount to managing symptoms of high estrogen. Although the effect of fasting *between* meals hasn't been formally studied, it is one of the most important management strategies for patients with any kind of IBS. In my clinic, the elimination of between-meal snacking is the single most effective, yet hardly known about strategy I use to counteract IBS. In fact, it is my first line strategy when trying to improve gut health for any reason, including when optimizing detoxification.

Taking a regular broad-spectrum prebiotic fiber is also essential for people with IBS, even though a low-residue (low fiber) diet may be a part of the initial treatment. It is a matter of trial and error to find the supplemental fibers that suit you. Since the explosion in research on the microbiome, there has also been an explosion in the number of prebiotic fiber supplements available on the market, so you have plenty of options to work with.

How long should I be on an Estrogen Clearing program?

The key to knowing whether the Estrogen Clearing Program has been a success for you is resolution of symptoms and an overall improvement in wellbeing. You can formalize the process of monitoring your symptoms using a questionnaire scoring system. In my practice, I use the Institute of Functional Medicine's 20-point questionnaire in addition to a specific women's health questionnaire. Depending on your response and the evolution of other health issues or hurdles, I recommend putting into practice both the Basic and Estrogen Clearing Programs for at least three months. After this time, I find many women have learnt how to tune in to their body's health and wellbeing. Over time, you will become an expert in personalizing your own program by dropping certain aspects and/or making diet/lifestyle additions while monitoring how you feel.

Can I do this program even though I'm highly stressed at the moment?

Although the Basic and Estrogen Clearing Programs can greatly improve your overall wellbeing, be aware that excessive stress is highly 'inflammatory' to your body and can reduce or cancel the effectiveness of any detoxification program. You will also be less able to 'tune in' to what things jive well with your body and what things don't.

The Solutions

The Progesterone Support Program

The Progesterone Support Program

As you now know from **Section One**, Progesterone is produced during the second half of the menstrual cycle, the *luteal phase*. In the *first* half of the cycle (follicular phase), and during cycles where no ovulation occurs, it is only produced in small amounts. As previously explained, *luteal phase* progesterone can fall slightly in your late 30s and 40s, and this fall may be responsible for some of the common symptoms at midlife. The Progesterone Support Program aims to address these progesterone-related symptoms in Zone 1, Zone 2, or Zone 3 women

Below is a list of symptoms that, if present, may indicate that you would benefit from the Progesterone Support Program. You may have these symptoms all through your menstrual cycle or confined to the last one to two weeks only.

If you have the following, consider the Progesterone Support Program:

- highly variable menstrual blood flow
- increase in menstrual blood clots and/or menstrual cramping
- increase in breast pain or tenderness
- midriff weight gain, swelling of extremities
- disturbed sleep, waking multiple times a night
- irritability, low mood, and low libido
- immune related issues like skin itchiness, rashes, joint pain, or autoimmunity.

The Progesterone Support Program involves:

- taking the steps in the Basic Program
- targeted nutritional supplements
- deeper focus on stress reduction
- vitex, an extract of the fruit called agnus-castus or chaste tree
- progesterone hormone therapy.

Nutritional supplements to support your body's progesterone

If you are still ovulating, a plentiful supply of *vitamin C* in food or whole food supplements may help improve your luteal phase progesterone levels.[380, 381] It has not been shown, however, to elevate progesterone levels high enough to be effective in infertility or to help support a pregnancy in women undergoing in-vitro fertilization.[382] Everyone's vitamin C requirements are different but you may have lower than optimal vitamin C if you have a diet devoid of fresh fruits and vegetables, have poor gut health (and therefore poor nutrient absorption), or have increased utilization of vitamin C stores through stress, infections, illness, poor sleep and smoking.[383, 384]

If you are on the go and live a high-stress life, you may benefit more from 'whole food vitamin C' supplements with bioflavonoids, especially if you eat packaged foods, fast foods, and leftovers on a regular basis. I favor whole food vitamin C with bioflavonoids in place of ascorbic acid alone, because bioflavonoids also have positive health effects on the heart, brain, skin, and immune system.[385] Foods rich in vitamin C include fresh herbs, bell peppers, tomatoes, broccoli, kale, blueberries, strawberries, and other dark berries. Many fruits other than berries are rich in vitamin C but have the disadvantage of being high in sugar. They include guavas, kiwifruit, oranges, lemons, and papaya. Be aware that all cooking processes reduce the vitamin C content of food. Choose shorter cooking times (<10 minutes) and lower temperatures (<160°F or 71°C) to help preserve it.

Another nutrient that may help optimize levels of progesterone is magnesium. Magnesium is a micro-nutrient or mineral that plays a vital role in many of the body's daily processes. It can be easily depleted through excessive stress and anything that increases oxidative stress in the body. In fact, one of the ways that magnesium could help progesterone levels is by reducing the physical body manifestations of excessive stress.[386-388] I often recommend at least 250 mg magnesium daily in the form of chelate, orotate, citrate, or bisglycinate. I also favor the slow-release formulations, especially for muscle or menstrual cramps, because as mentioned previously, high levels taken all at once can be rapidly removed by your kidneys. Check with your health provider that you don't have any kidney problems before taking magnesium supplements.

More reasons to focus on reducing stress

When you are stressed, your body produces a higher amount of the stress hormone called cortisol (or cortisone). Excess cortisol in the body can reduce the ability of your corpus luteum to produce progesterone during the luteal phase.[389] It can also reduce progesterone's positive effects on the body. We know that women who are suffering from severe stress (e.g., have a history of sexual abuse) are more likely to suffer from premenstrual tension (PMT) symptoms, a disorder that has been linked to a faster fall in progesterone at the end of the menstrual cycle.[112, 390]

Stress reduction strategies, such as the morning color-breathing and stretching routines outlined in the Basic Program, have many health benefits. Given the specific effect stress can have on progesterone, if you have symptoms that appear to be low progesterone-related, you may wish to consider additional stress-reduction activities. Examples include mindfulness meditation, cognitive behavioral therapy, belly breathing, yoga, or even qi gong, all of which have been shown to be effective stress reducing strategies.[300, 391, 392]

What about drinking coffee and stress? While I am the first person to recommend 1-2 good quality sugarless coffees in the morning, there are a handful of caffeine-sensitive people who can get too activated after drinking coffee. If you are severely stressed and not sleeping well, aim to limit your coffee intake to a single cup once a day before 10 am. Even a small amount of residual caffeine in your bloodstream (e.g., 12 hours after a strong coffee) may reduce your rest and digest bodily functions and reduce the quality of your sleep. If you have caffeine in your bloodstream when you go to bed, your beneficial slow-wave sleep is reduced and the less beneficial arousal times are increased without you realizing it.[393] The deleterious effect on sleep is also more pronounced after our 40s and this, in turn, can adversely affect proges-terone production.

Vitex: Agnus-castus or chaste tree fruit

Vitex is the abbreviation for *Vitex rotundifolia*. It is a fruit extract also known as 'agnus castus' or chaste tree fruit. Vitex contains numerous plant compounds, the most well-known being casticin, luteolin, rotundifuran, and agnuside. It has been used medicinally for at least 2,000 years and has been extensively studied in at least 50 women's health studies in Europe and the UK, where it is used widely.[394] It has an excellent safety profile and is approved for use in Europe for a number of women's health issues, including menstrual irregularities,[395] mastalgia[395] and PMT.[396] I have been using it in my practice for some years now and the beneficial effects in my patients are completely in alignment with the positive results seen in the research studies.[394]

Vitex has been shown to help reduce symptoms linked to low progester-one including menstrual cramping, PMT, mastalgia, and irritability.[397] It has been shown to help regulate menstrual cycles in young women, but it hasn't been studied specifically in midlife women with menstrual irregularities.[398] In my experience, it doesn't help regulate the menstrual irregularities seen in Zone 2 and Zone 3 women, but it does help reduce the mastalgia and severe PMT symptoms that I see frequently in these Zones.

The beneficial actions of Vitex likely relate to its effects on both the estrogen and progesterone *receptors*, and overall, it favors an increase in the actions of progesterone in the body. It also has a mild blocking or 'regulating' action on two important brain chemicals called dopamine and prolactin, thereby helping reduce the hormonal upheavals produced by life stressors.[399] By way of its effects on the dopamine receptors, it has been shown to lower the pituitary hormones FSH and LH, potentially promoting an estrogen-calming effect that would be helpful in Zone 1 and Zone 2 women.[400] Vitex also seems to be a strong antioxidant and anti-inflammatory agent.[401] The anti-inflammatory effects have been shown to be mediated via suppression of several 'inflammatory cytokine' molecules and via reduction in levels of tumor-necrosis factor (TNF-alpha).[402, 403] All these properties seem to make vitex a designer food extract for midlife women.

Vitex is easy to take orally once or twice a day with very few women reporting any side effects. In a few women however, it can apparently cause nausea, headache, loose bowels, mild acne, itch, or a rash.[404] If you are on any hormone therapy, the oral contraceptive pill or other medication, check with your healthcare provider that it is compatible. If you are a small-build woman or tend to react to new foods or supplements, start with a lower dose of 250 mg daily. Otherwise, you can start with 500 mg and then if all is well after a few weeks, you can increase the dose to 1000-1500 mg daily, the target dose for most women. Beneficial effects can take 2-3 months to become apparent, so I will often have women take it for at least 3 months before deciding whether or not it has been helpful.

Progesterone hormone therapy

If your symptoms are not relieved with the Basic Program, targeted nutritional supplements and consistent stress reduction techniques, you may want to talk to your healthcare provider about progesterone therapy. Progesterone and its synthetic versions (progestins) have been used to treat heavy and irregular bleeding in midlife women for decades.[405] However, little is known or has been studied regarding its use in non-menstrual symptoms such as bloating, headache, mastalgia, hand/feet swelling, disturbed sleep and low mood/libido. Although these symptoms are recognized as part of the premenstrual syndrome (PMS), they are not recognized as increasingly common in midlife women. There are no clinical studies examining a possible link between midlife symptoms and a fall in luteal phase progesterone, but studies in younger women with PMT suggest there may be a link.[135, 406]

Premenstrual symptoms are traditionally treated with birth control pills or synthetic progestins, and while these can alleviate symptoms in a few women, they are often not effective, can have adverse health effects such as blood clotting, and can trigger a worsening of symptoms such as bloating, irritability and breast pain.[407-409] Synthetic progestins include norethisterone, levonorgestrel (the progestin delivered by the Mirena® IUD) and etonogestrel (delivered by the implanted contraception called Implanon®), and all the progestins used in birth control pills. Birth control pills have an advantage in that they provide effective contraception if it is needed. Even after the age of 40, risk of pregnancy must always be a consideration. In my practice, I rarely need to resort to prescribing birth control pills or synthetic progestins for symptom relief in midlife women because the strategies within the Basic, Estrogen Clearing, and Progesterone Support Programs are effective in most women as well as being health-promoting. In addition, I find an increasing number of women want information about what they can do to help themselves rather than take another pill.

Because of natural progesterone's excellent safety profile, I nearly always use it in place of synthetic progestins.[410] I use high-dose oral progesterone (300-400 mg) for heavy bleeding and usual-dose progesterone (100-200 mg) for premenstrual symptoms. Because clinical research information on progesterone in midlife symptoms is virtually absent, I always prescribe it on a trial basis and if it has not been effective or there are unwanted side effects, I make sure it is discontinued after a 3-6-month trial.

Progesterone therapy according to your Zone

Progesterone therapy is administered in either a capsule or, less commonly, a cream. The progesterone used in the capsules and creams is manufactured from a plant compound called *diosgenin*. The only available pharmaceutical progesterone preparations are 100 or 200 mg tablets. Compounding pharmacists can prepare progesterone capsules, troches or creams in individualized doses that can be adjusted based on your needs and your healthcare practitioner's assessment. All oral tablets or capsules should contain 'micronized' progesterone to improve its absorption in the gut. When a medication is micronized, it is broken down into 'micro' particles and suspended in oil. NOTE: progesterone tablets should be taken *before bed*, because firstly they can cause daytime sleepiness, and secondly, they benefit sleep.[411]

Oral progesterone suggestions to discuss with your healthcare provider:

Zone 1: 100-200 mg oral progesterone on cycle-day 14 and continue until you start a menstrual period. This is known as supplemental luteal phase or 'cyclical' progesterone therapy.

Zone 2: if you have very irregular short and long menstrual cycles, you can't be sure when your luteal phase is, so simply start 100-200 mg oral progesterone on or around cycle-day 10 and stop it as soon as your menstrual period starts. If you are bleeding heavily and/or for more than 14 days, see your healthcare provider about taking a higher dose of the progesterone or other medical treatments.

Zone 3: again, like in Zone 2, if you have irregular cycles with long gaps between periods, you won't be able to know when your luteal phase is. Simply start 100-200 mg oral progesterone on or around cycle-day 10 and stop it as soon as your menstrual period starts. Being in Zone 3, there is always a chance that your current menstrual period will be your last. If you reach the 6-month mark of taking progesterone without a menstrual period, talk to your healthcare provider about continuing the progesterone, and about treating other menopausal symptoms should they arise.

Zone 4: in this Zone, progesterone is usually prescribed with estrogen as part of *menopausal hormone therapy* or *MHT*. It is taken either continuously or for about 14 days a month. Breakthrough spotting or light bleeding with MHT is less likely with higher doses (200 mg) and when taken continuously rather than for just 14 days a month.

Progesterone cream

In my clinical experience, cyclical progesterone cream can be very effective for women with symptoms of low progesterone in Zone 1, Zone 2 and Zone 3. Unfortunately, there have been no large clinical trials to assess its efficacy, and there likely won't be in future because there are currently no commercially available pharmaceutical versions. There were a number of studies at least 20 years ago that showed that applying progesterone cream didn't lead to any increase in the blood levels of progesterone even at high doses[412] and didn't seem to benefit bone, hot flushes or mood.[413] Because of the lack of rise in blood levels seen in most studies, it has been concluded that progesterone creams would not be sufficient to protect the endometrium from the effects of estrogen. Despite this, progesterone cream has remained popular, and I can certainly attest to the fact that in many women, it seems to have a highly beneficial effect.

It is possible that a measurable rise in blood levels of progesterone is not required for its beneficial effects. In fact, well-known hormone biochemist Dr. Stanczyk found that applying progesterone cream led to a rise in progesterone levels within the small, local capillaries.[414] He surmised that the progesterone in the cream moved into the subcutaneous fat under the skin, then into the capillaries. Once in the capillaries, rather than being transported to the larger blood vessels, the progesterone then moves into the lymphatic circulation, and then into other body tissues including the salivary glands, the endometrium, and brain. These findings were duplicated in another small study of ten menopausal women showing that after application of progesterone cream, progesterone levels rise 10-fold and 100-fold in the capillaries and saliva respectively.[415] This study also found that progesterone gel was absorbed similarly to cream, raising both capillary and saliva levels of progesterone. These findings seem to explain why so many midlife women feel its positive effects, especially when their progesterone levels start to wane in late reproductive age and perimenopause.

Given the absence of significant clinical studies on progesterone cream and the fact that is not a commercially viable product for pharmaceutical companies, it is not and will likely never be an 'approved therapy' for women. So, if practitioners want to prescribe progesterone cream, they need to prescribe a compounded version and be aware they are prescribing it as an 'off-label' (outside of approved use) medication. Although its safety cannot be fully assessed outside of clinical trials, a reasonable level of safety can be implied from existing studies on *oral* progesterone. I believe it is reasonable for health practitioners to prescribe progesterone cream for low-progesterone symptoms for women in Zone 1, Zone 2 and Zone 3, but not for endometrial protection which requires oral progesterone. I will outline how I prescribe it on **page 182**.

What about intra-vaginal progesterone cream or pessaries?

I reserve vaginal progesterone cream or pessaries for severe bleeding disorders in women who cannot tolerate high-dose oral formulations. Intravaginal progesterone delivers high levels of progesterone to the endometrium and uterus, and so can be used to protect the endometrium when taking estrogen therapy in menopause. Consult your healthcare provider about this.

The Solutions

Targeted Solutions (1):

- Heavy menstrual bleeding
- Endometriosis and adenomyosis
- Fibroids
- Hysterectomy for the management of fibroids

Heavy menstrual bleeding

As discussed in **Section One**, heavy bleeding can become a problem in some women at midlife due to changes in estrogen and progesterone levels. If you think your periods have become heavier, you can use the criteria on **page 40** or some of the indicators below to determine if you have what your healthcare provider would consider 'heavy menstrual bleeding'.

If you have the following, you have heavy menstrual bleeding:

- soak at least 15 medium pads during an entire period OR
- soak at least 8 super-size pads during an entire period OR
- soak at least 10 super-size tampons during an entire period OR
- fill 3 or more menstrual cups during an entire period (80-90 mL or ~3 fl.oz.).

If you think you meet the criteria for heavy menstrual bleeding or you are concerned about how much you are bleeding, you should arrange to see your healthcare provider. In the meantime, you can start using the Basic and Estrogen Clearing Programs, which together help counteract any aggravating effect that inflammation and/or high estrogen may be having on your menstrual blood loss.

When you consult your healthcare provider, take a diary or a completed menstrual cycle app to your appointment to show them estimates of the number of pads and tampons you need throughout a menstrual period. Include a description of the number and size of any clots that you see as well. In terms of investigating related problems, make sure you ask them whether you need a blood test to check for blood loss anemia, iron-deficiency or even inherited clotting disorders. In terms of investigating underlying structural causes, ask whether you should have an ultrasound of your uterus to exclude issues like fibroids and adenomyosis.

Tips you can try at home for heavy bleeding and period pain:

- Use the Basic and Estrogen Clearing Programs.
- 200-400 mg ibuprofen[416] every 4-5 hours with food during the first 1-3 days of heavy bleeding.
- If moderate-severe pain, add 500 mg paracetamol/acetaminophen to ibuprofen.
- Keep well hydrated and include an electrolyte drink, especially in hot weather.
- Add turmeric to your curries or take a 500-1000 mg turmeric supplement.
- 3 mg boron[417] tablets 2-3 times daily from 3 days before your period starts to the final day of your period.

Treatment suggestions to discuss with your healthcare provider:

- 100-150 mg oral progesterone (micronized) for excess clots.
- Tranexamic acid on the first 1-3 days of a heavy bleeding.
- Progestin-delivering intra-uterine devices (IUD).
- As a last resort, surgery, including endometrial ablation or hysterectomy.
- If you have menstrual bleeding in the setting of chronic illness, excess fatigue, unexplained aches/pains and/or poor gut function, you may benefit from medications that treat mast cell activation disorders (e.g., MCAS[211]).

Heavy menstrual bleeding in Zone 2 or Zone 3

Menstrual bleeding can become excessive in Zone 2 and Zone 3 when menstrual cycles become irregular and unpredictable. As a result, you can be caught off-guard with sudden excessive bleeding called 'flooding'. When patients are in this predicament, I use high-dose continuous progesterone capsules (300-400 mg daily) or synthetic progestin norethisterone tablets (10-15 mg daily). Neither high-dose progesterone or norethisterone will restore normality to your irregular menstrual cycles, but when used continuously for several months, they can greatly reduce bleeding until your menstrual cycles settle.[418]

If your heavy bleeding is likely to continue past six months or so, you should discuss other options such as a progestin-releasing IUD (e.g., Mirena), endometrial ablation or hysterectomy with your healthcare provider. An endometrial ablation is a straightforward surgical procedure which is effective at abolishing heavy menstrual bleeding but is only suitable if there are minimal structural issues like fibroids. [419] In addition, it has a 15-20% failure rate requiring further medical treatment or hysterectomy.[420]

If you have ongoing flooding or continuous heavy bleeding, ask your healthcare provider about:

- 300-400 mg (high dose) continuous oral progesterone before bed
- 10-15 mg (high dose) continuous norethisterone daily
- birth control pills (needs discussion of possible side effects)
- levonorgestrel-releasing intrauterine system (Mirena®)
- endometrial ablation
- hysterectomy.

In the past, most women with uncontrolled menstrual bleeding at midlife had to have a hysterectomy (surgical removal of their uterus). Although this procedure can be an absolute 'gift' for some women with severe, painful and heavy periods, with the invention of effective treatments like endometrial ablation and the levonorgestrel-releasing intrauterine system, the need for hysterectomies has fallen somewhat. According to a Veterans Affairs study between 2008 and 2014, the rate of hysterectomy in the U.S. fell from 4 to 2.6 per 1,000 women.[421] A similar trend in the reduction of hysterectomies has been seen in Portugal, and in Australia where rates have fallen from around 8 per 1,000 between 2000 and 2009, to about 4.7 per 1,000 between 2010 and 2016.[422]

Endometriosis and adenomyosis

Both endometriosis and adenomyosis can cause severe pain and heavy bleeding. They are similar conditions in that they are associated with marked inflammation in the uterus, irritable bowel syndrome, and autoimmune conditions.

Excess estrogen may also play a role but to a lesser degree. When severe and not relieved by the combined Basic and Estrogen Clearing Programs, they need surgical intervention, but a number of natural anti-inflammatory agents have recently been investigated including resveratrol and melatonin.

Fibroids

Between 70 and 80% of women have a uterine fibroid, but only a third know that they have one, or have any heavy bleeding and/or pain because of one.[54] Compared to endometriosis and adenomyosis, fibroids are more about counteracting excess estrogen than excess inflammation, although both factors are involved.[423] If you know you have one or more fibroids, chances are you will have had a trans-vaginal ultrasound scan outlining how many and what size they are. You may have also been told you can watch and wait to see if they worsen, or that they will need surgical treatment.

In general, if your fibroids become an issue when in Zone 1 or Zone 2, they are likely to worsen before they get better after menopause. Nevertheless, the Basic and Estrogen Clearing Programs may be able to help slow their growth and thus reduce their effect on menstrual bleeding and pain.

If your fibroids become an issue in Zone 3, they may also worsen, but your symptoms are more likely to improve after using the Basic and Estrogen Clearing Programs, because your estrogen levels will be starting to drop anyway.

If your fibroids are a problem in Zone 4 and beyond, they are less likely to worsen unless you need to take high-dose estrogen as part of menopausal hormone therapy. In this case, they may need to be monitored and/or treated.

Some cases of fibroids cannot be dealt with adequately without surgery or anti-estrogen medical therapy so, if you are concerned, discuss these options with your healthcare provider.

Steps you can take while deciding on going ahead with surgery for endometriosis, adenomyosis or fibroids:

- use the Basic and Estrogen Clearing Programs
- low-histamine diet to calm excessive immune system reactivity and excessive mast cell activity
- 400 mg ibuprofen every 4-5 hours with food during the first 1-3 days of heavy bleeding
- if moderate-severe pain, add 500 mg paracetamol/acetaminophen to ibuprofen
- explore anti-inflammatory herbals[425] like curcumin, resveratrol, quercetin, and berberine
- de-stress as much as possible to encourage your rest and digest functions
- avoid foods high in nickel.[424]

Hysterectomy for the management of fibroids

The management of large bulky fibroids that affect so many women has developed over the last five decades, and there have been some improvements in the surgical and other techniques that can shrink or remove the fibroids themselves without removing the whole uterus.[426] You may be one of those women who are more than happy to have 'the whole lot' removed because of the pain and suffering it has caused. You wouldn't have anything to worry about anymore, right? Perhaps, but having a hysterectomy is not without risk and can often cause other little-known side effects. The usual risks of having a hysterectomy include excess bleeding during surgery and then following surgery, wound infection (1-5%), internal or external wound breakdown (2-3%), deep vein thrombosis, lung clots, nerve injury (0.5-2%) and intraoperative injury to the gut or bladder (1-2%).[427] The surgeons involved usually talk about these prior to surgery, but most don't discuss some of the longer-term, lesser-known side effects.

Lesser-known side effects of a hysterectomy

Other side effects from having a hysterectomy have to do with the inevitable and sometimes substantial changes that occur to the internal structure of your pelvis, bladder function, and sexual function. Because the uterus is an integral part of the pelvis along with the bladder, the bowel, ovaries, arteries, veins, lymphatics, etc., its position and structure form an integral part of the 'scaffolding' that holds all the contents of the pelvis together. When the bulk of this 'pelvic scaffolding' is removed, the 'scaffolding' is considerably weakened and other pelvic contents, including the small bowel, the bladder, and rectum, 'fall in' to where the uterus was. This is likely to explain some of the chronic pelvic pain that up to 10% of women complain of after this surgery.[428]

If you have a hysterectomy and you also had one or more vaginal births, the added birth canal trauma can increase risk of urine incontinence even further, something that can occur months or years down the track.[429] For a few women however, removing a problematic bulky uterus can actually improve incontinence in the short term. What about sexual function? For some women, removing the source of pain and heavy bleeding can increase sexual activity/functioning. But depending on you as an individual and any damage suffered during surgery, after having a hysterectomy you may get pain on intercourse, reduced sensation on intercourse, reduced vaginal lubrication, and reduced ability to have an orgasm.[430]

The intricacies of sexual function after hysterectomy are too large a subject for this book but I think many of us would find it interesting to learn how the vagina, cervix, and uterus 'behave' during sexual intercourse.[431] Jenny Higgins of Wisconsin University says, 'The uterus is involved in orgasm. It moves up, it balloons, it contracts, it causes the vagina to tent (an activity aided by the broad ligaments within the pelvis). The broad ligaments swell and tighten, and draw up the vagina, lengthening it.' I think many of you who are in tune with your bodies, or who have felt 'internal' orgasms (as opposed to clitoral orgasms) may resonate with this. You could perhaps also understand how challenging this would be to study! It would be no small task to make sense of hundreds of women's accounts of their orgasmic experiences either before or after hysterectomy.

The Solutions

Targeted Solutions (2):

- PMS or PMT and related symptoms (Premenstrual syndrome or premenstrual tension)
  - Headache in PMS
  - Mastalgia, breast soreness
  - Abdominal bloating, excess midriff weight
  - Swelling of the extremities
  - Anger and irritability
  - Low mood, depression and anxiety
- Disturbed sleep
- Brain health
- Heart health
- Libido
- Bone health, exercise and vitamin D
- Thyroid and autoimmunity

PMS or PMT related symptoms

PMS can occur at any age, but some studies suggest it gets more common towards menopause. PMS severely affects 5-10% women and mildly affects about 30%.[432] The severe mood disorder linked to PMS called PMDD (premenstrual dysphoria disorder) often requires antidepressant therapy.[132] Other common PMS symptoms listed below have not been definitively studied, so little is known about their underlying cause and effective treatments. Many women with severe PMS are given a trial of birth control pills, but these can worsen symptoms or cause unpleasant side effects in some women, and they come with more risks over the age of 40.

Common PMS symptoms:

- headache
- mastalgia or breast soreness
- abdominal bloating, swelling of extremities
- anger, irritability, mood swings
- low mood, depression, feeling overwhelmed, emotional, and/or teary.

Although these symptoms are recognized as being 'premenstrual', they can also occur throughout the menstrual cycle. I find most of these symptoms can be relieved using functional medicine principles, even when accompanied by depression requiring antidepressant therapy. The Basic and Progesterone Support programs underpin management of PMS, and where appropriate, I also trial progesterone cream.

Progesterone cream for PMS

Although there are no approved indications for progesterone cream, over the years, I have come across many midlife patients with PMS who have either already had a positive experience with it or wanted to try it. Because of this and my extensive experience with prescribing oral forms of progesterone, I began prescribing progesterone cream off-label for PMS. As I have explained on **page 170**, the benefits of progesterone cream in midlife women have yet to be formally studied and so the reasons why it can benefit women, particularly those with PMS, are not well understood.[412] Although there are no clinical data on the efficacy and safety of progesterone *cream*, we know progesterone itself has an excellent safety profile when given for luteal phase support or as part of menopausal hormone therapy.[433]

You should discuss the various options with your healthcare provider, but the usual dose for progesterone cream for PMS is 0.5 mL of a 2.5-5% cream applied daily to the inside of the thigh/upper arm or back of neck between cycle-day 7-14 and the start of your next menstrual period. The longer you have PMS symptoms prior to a menstrual period, the earlier in your cycle you can start it. Because the need for progesterone cream changes over time and through the menopause transition, I always recommend trying to stop it every 6-12 months, to see whether the symptoms have improved. If you have been using the Basic and Progesterone Support Programs for 6-12 months, your symptoms may be sufficiently controlled without the use of progesterone cream.

If your PMS symptoms include disturbed sleep, I would also add 150-200 mg *oral* progesterone taken before bed. You can use this with progesterone cream or on its own. Always stop the oral progesterone when you start a menstrual bleed, so your endometrium can fully shed as usual. Vaginal and rectal formulations of progesterone are available, but these are usually only needed in fertility situations when very high levels of progesterone are required to maintain a pregnancy.

Headache in PMS

Although there are many underlying contributors to headache and migraine, if your headache/migraine started in your late 30s to 40s, it could be triggered or worsened by a rise in estrogen at midlife. If this is you, it may be worth trying a combination of the Basic and Estrogen Clearing Programs. If your headache/migraine started after reaching Zone 3 or Zone 4, your headache is more likely due low estrogen rather than high estrogen and may be relieved with menopausal hormone therapy.

Mastalgia, breast soreness

Most women have some degree of breast soreness, especially during the few days or week prior to a menstrual period. Many women have 'movement pain', which is when their pain worsens during activity or exercise. In some women, this can be reduced by wearing a sport-grade supportive bra, but in others, their breast soreness is so severe they cannot tolerate wearing a bra at all. Thankfully, I find these problems can be substantially relieved with both the Basic and Estrogen Clearing Programs in addition to vitex (a supplement made from a fruit extract) from a reliable organic source. The starting dose for vitex is 250-500 mg daily, increasing to a target dose of 1000-1500 mg daily over a week or so. You should take vitex for at least three months to see whether you benefit from it or not. It has been found in multiple studies to be an effective and safe intervention for breast soreness, but I find it to be even more effective when women also follow the Basic and Estrogen Clearing Programs.

If your breast soreness accompanies lumpy or 'cystic' breasts, be sure to get a urine iodine test done to check your body's iodine levels (it is measured with a single-time morning urine sample). Low iodine has been linked to cystic breasts, increased risk of breast cancer and other health problems.[434] If your urine iodine is low, you can increase your iodine levels by using iodized salt and eating iodine-rich foods like shellfish, fish (especially cod), liver, black-eyed peas, and dried seaweed. Lesser amounts of iodine come from eggs, prunes, yoghurt, hard cheeses, kidney beans, potatoes (from iodine rich soils), berries, bananas, and other fruits and vegetables. Some women need to take a supplement because diet sources are not sufficient or because dietary preferences result in suboptimal nutritional intake. If this is you, ask your healthcare provider to guide you through taking an iodine supplement. Once you start a supplement, have them check your iodine levels on a semiregular basis, especially if you have had an over- or under-active thyroid.

Abdominal bloating, excess midriff weight

As discussed in **Section Two**, I have found many midlife women complain of abdominal bloating, discomfort, and an expanding waistline. The contributors to this problem can be addressed by undertaking the steps in the Basic and Estrogen Clearing Programs. If you have this issue, pay particular attention to strengthening your digestion and elimination and include digestive bitters (**page 151**; dandelion, solidago, gentian, Oregon grape, etc.) with your main meals. If constipation remains an issue after these steps, re-focus on de-stressing techniques and fiber supplements. If abdominal pain, flatulence and/or diarrhea are an issue, ask your healthcare provider about getting tested for coeliac disease. If bloating seems to be related to what you eat, try eliminating all gluten-containing grains. If you are also carrying excess weight, aim to eliminate both gluten and non-gluten containing grains (this includes corn and peanuts) until you are at, or near, your ideal weight. If you go on a gluten-free or grain-free eating plan, make sure you include a selection of supplemental fibers on a daily basis to replace the fiber you're not eating with whole grains.

Stubborn or severe abdominal bloating

If you have ongoing bloating after using digestive bitters, eliminating gluten grains, and/or trying a grain-free diet, you may want to try reducing or eliminating foods that contain high amounts of FODMAPs or *fermentable oligosaccharides, disaccharides, monosaccharides and polyols.* These foods can cause abdominal discomfort by distending the gut with excess gas. Foods high in FODMAPs include the brassica vegetables (broccoli, cauliflower, brussels sprouts), artichoke, leek, onion, garlic, wholegrain breads, legumes, pulses, wheat pasta, rye, cashews, pistachios, apples, pears, mangoes, and high fructose corn syrup. You can search for a more exhaustive list online and explore the now readily available low-FODMAP recipe books.

Although a low-FODMAP diet is a very popular 'go-to' for irritable bowel symptoms (IBS), over time, FODMAP diet restrictions can substantially reduce beneficial bowel flora because high-FODMAP foods contain healthy fiber which feeds and maintains healthy bowel bacteria. Therefore, after about three months of restricting the FODMAPs, you should try slowly reintroducing them, one FODMAP food at a time. If your symptoms return after reintroducing only a few FODMAPs in small amounts, you should ask your healthcare provider to investigate underlying *causes* for your bloating.

One common but under-appreciated cause is retention of stool or constipation with large bowel fecal loading. Most people have no idea that they have fecal overloading because they have 'a bowel motion everyday'. If you have frequent or occasional hard stools or you have alternating loose and hard stools, you may have fecal overloading. A less common cause is SIBO or *small intestinal bacterial overgrowth* which I discussed on **pages 57–59**. Both fecal overloading and SIBO can cause uncomfortable or painful upper abdominal bloating within 30-60 minutes after a meal, and this may last several hours.

If this is you, the first action to take is to ask your healthcare provider to request a simple abdominal X-ray to exclude fecal overloading. If you have significant fecal overloading, you should see your healthcare provider about starting an aperient program and investigate which foods may be triggering it. I have found 'silent' fecal overloading (no symptoms) to be extremely common with some of the more common foods causing it being gluten-containing breads/cookies and some dairy products like mature cheese.

Options for the management of fecal overloading:

- once-twice daily osmotic laxative (draws liquid into the bowel)
- magnesium citrate and/or oxide before bed
- drink pure water (1-1.5 L daily)
- use stool softeners (like docusate) in preference to stimulants
- only use stimulants like bisacodyl and sennosides intermittently
- monitor your progress regularly using abdominal X-rays
- if your progress is slow, consider asking your healthcare provider about cleaning colonic procedures
- introduce prebiotic fibers like psyllium *after* resolution of your symptoms and when your fecal overloading has mostly cleared.

If you don't have any signs of fecal overloading, you may have SIBO or another less common condition. Be aware that SIBO breath-testing investigations are notoriously unreliable but can be helpful as a one-off initial investigation in some settings. Avoid healthcare providers who order *repeated* SIBO testing, especially if they say, 'it is to monitor your progress'. The unreliability of SIBO testing does not warrant the cost involved and results are often mis-interpreted. Instead, seek out a healthcare provider who is experienced in the management of SIBO and who uses your symptoms as a guide to treatment. They should also be well-versed in how to promote gut health and how to help maintain the health of your microbiome.

Swelling of extremities (hands, feet, limbs)

Provided you are otherwise healthy, have no heart problems and baseline blood testing has been checked by your healthcare provider, I suggest focusing on the Basic Program for this problem. If symptoms persist or only partly resolve, add in the steps from the Estrogen Clearing Program. Swelling can also respond well to progesterone cream, whether the swelling is constant or cyclical and part of PMS. I have women apply 0.5 mL 2.5-5% progesterone cream on the inside of the arm/thigh or the back of the neck every night except the *first* 10 days of a menstrual cycle. A trial of about three months should be sufficient to determine whether it is useful or not in reducing the swelling.

Anger and irritability

I found the women in my Ph.D. study reported unexpected outbursts of anger, particularly those in Zones 1, 2, and 3. Many women will also say they think their 'bodies are starting to change' but cannot pinpoint whether this is why they feel angry. We don't understand why women feel more 'edgy' at midlife, but it could relate to the slight upshift in androgens that can occur in addition to the changes in estrogen and progesterone.[435] Midlife is also the time when many women are completing their roles as homemakers and child-bearers, and now have an opportunity to 'come back to themselves'. Perhaps many of us feel like 'hitting out' because we no longer feel the need to cater to those around us.

Perhaps this has something to do with a change in the hormonal ebb and flows. For example, we may suddenly become aware of the injustices we have lived through or simply the fact that we 'lost ourselves' by putting others first for so many years. Using the Basic and Estrogen Clearing Programs can help stabilize intense emotions by reducing swings in blood sugar, improving gut-brain health, and helping reduce the high kick-ups in estrogen.

Tips to help manage outbursts of anger:

- eat only fresh foods and reduce stress (Basic Program)
- include color-breathing and stretching daily (**page 125-129**)
- if high estrogen symptoms, use the Estrogen Clearing Program
- if low estrogen symptoms, see your healthcare provider about hormone therapy
- request a sleep study if you are known to snore
- try doing a gratitude diary, especially before sleep
- if you have an overwhelming schedule, aim to make it more manageable
- explore any unresolved emotional issues with an experienced professional.

Low mood and depression

Depression should be treated seriously, so don't delay in seeing your health-care provider to access the appropriate counselling and medication if needed. I don't often initiate antidepressant medication because my patients are either stabilized and happy on their medication or want help to get off them to trial other therapies. With or without antidepressant medication, the steps you can take to improve low mood relate to addressing hormonal upheavals consistent with your Zone, and to addressing gut health and inflammation.

Why address gut health to improve your mood? Because mood chemicals in the gut and brain are intimately connected via the nervous system and the gut flora.[436] This connection has become increasingly recognized and has been referred to as the gut-brain axis and I discuss this at length on **pages 73-77**.[437] Research has shown us that inflammation in the gut is linked to inflammation in the brain or neuroinflammation.[438]

Tips for low mood and depression:

- reduce whole-body inflammation (Basic Program)
- exercise regularly and include some intense exercise
- reduce alcohol to 1-2 standard drinks twice a week or less
- request a sleep study to exclude sleep apnea if you snore
- ask about hormone therapy if you think you have low estrogen symptoms
- try 1000-1500 mg vitex fruit extract daily for 3-4 months.

If you can do the Basic Program for at least three months, you should be able to determine whether it is effective in helping your mood. If you get partial improvement, keep going with the Basic program and consider adding in other treatments. Some women with low mood also benefit from nutritional supplements including those that provide methylation support (e.g., S-adenosyl-L-methionine or SAMe), or herbal preparations like St John's Wort.

Anxiety

Midlife for women is often a time of upheavals in careers, relationships and family life and if we become anxious, we often know what it is about. Talking over your situational issues with someone can often alleviate anxiety and allow you to form a strategy to amend or improve your situation. Sometimes, however, we can get very anxious for no apparent reason. This may be a result of the increased hormonal fluctuations characteristic of midlife and in some cases may be amenable to estrogen therapy.[439] I have also found 3-5% progesterone cream applied to the neck every night except from cycle day 1-10 is very helpful. Discuss these options with your healthcare provider.

Ashwagandha can also be helpful in some women (500-1000 mg 3-4 times a day). Be aware however that while some women greatly benefit from it, others don't seem to respond at all. In some women, a simple magnesium supplement (e.g., 500 mg magnesium bisglycinate or magnesium chelate) can help them relax. Whatever supplement you try, a 2-3-month trial is usually long enough to determine whether it is effective or not, but sometimes you may need to stop them and then restart them to find out.

Tips for anxiety:

- reach out to a trusted friend or therapist to 'talk it over'
- reduce excess stress (Basic Program)
- include color-breathing and stretching daily (**pages 125-129**)
- favor more gentle forms of exercise
- ensure you get adequate quality sleep
- see your healthcare provider about medications including estrogen therapy or progesterone cream.

Mycotoxin illness, a lesser-known cause of anxiety

One under-recognized disorder called mycotoxin illness or mold-related illness is an important cause of adult-onset anxiety and when recognized, can be managed and reversed. The anxiety is often described as being severe and 'out of nowhere'. As I mentioned on **page 138**, mycotoxins are naturally occurring estrogen-like toxins produced by mold that are classed as *xenoestrogens*. Mycotoxin illness is caused by exposure to excessive amounts of mycotoxins within water-damaged buildings. The illness involves the direct effect of myco-toxins on the body in addition to the excess whole-body *inflammation* that results from the toxins. It is not just a mold allergy, but it isn't a mold *infection* either. Although allergic symptoms can be an aspect of mycotoxin illness, it is mostly characterized by systemic inflammatory symptoms including fatigue, fleeting rashes, headaches, joint aches, and brain fog. This is why it is also often referred to as chronic inflammatory response syndrome or CIRS.

If you have new-onset anxiety that is severe, is out of character for you or doesn't seem to respond to treatment, ask yourself whether you may have mold-related illness. Then ask yourself whether your home or office is or has been water-damaged. Water damage can occur because of flooding, ceiling leaks, water-pipe damage, excess condensation or lack of airflow in damp environ-ments. The most common causes of water-damage that I see in my practice are hidden bathroom pipe/shower leaks and air-conditioning leaks including poorly designed condensation management. In a water-damaged building, you will often smell unpleasant 'mustiness', especially if the building is closed for days to weeks. Some of the worst affected buildings don't have any visible mold, but if you see mold growing on numerous pieces of furniture and/or your clothes and shoes, you do need to consider whether you have significant amounts of mold growing in the walls or ceiling. Once water damage has occurred in a building, mold continues to be a problem long after the offending leak has been rectified, especially in humid environments. You can find more information about mold-related illness and water-damaged buildings at: <//iseai.org/resources/>.

Because mycotoxins are xenoestrogens, being exposed to high amounts of mycotoxins may be particularly problematic for midlife women. When dealing with more erratic and sometimes higher hormone levels, especially estrogen, midlife women may have increased risk of getting mold-related toxicity symptoms and inflammation. If you want to be assessed for mold-related illness, consult a healthcare provider who is knowledgeable about it (see www.iseasi.org). Remember that mold-related illness is *not* an infection but rather is an inflammatory illness that results from excess mold growth *inside* the walls of a building. It is a little-known illness that is gaining more attention, but you will still be able to find a handful of publications from immunology and infectious diseases specialists who argue that it doesn't exist. These specialists have likely never seen or treated patients with mold-related illness. It certainly does exist.

The most important 'treatment' in mold-related illness is removing yourself from the building that is the source of your excess mycotoxin exposure. The practicalities of this can be a nightmare, so it is important to get a building inspection from a professional who is experienced in water damage and house mold. While it can be annoying to find significant amounts of mold in the walls of your home, it is worth addressing because it can be devastating to your health. Another important thing to remember about mold-related illness is that while mycotoxins adversely affect everyone's health by causing inflamma-tion, only some people become extremely unwell, get severely anxious and/or debilitated. In other words, there are individual factors involved as far as which members of a large household get sick from the same water-damaged home.

Disturbed sleep

Many of us look back to our younger days when our head hit the pillow and we would be 'out like a light' for eight or nine hours. For some midlife women, sleep disturbance starts in Zone 1 and continues, but for others it starts later in Zone 4. Either way, it is likely that hormonal factors contribute to the disturbance. Although we do not know the exact mechanisms, the midlife hormonal changes likely lead to changes in the hypothalamus, in the center of our brain. The hypothalamus controls all the automatic functions in the body like breathing, excretion, digestion, sweating and sleep. It regulates our circadian rhythm and the balance between rapid-eye movement (REM) and non-REM sleep.[440]

Our natural sleep rhythm involves cycling through light sleep, REM sleep and non-REM sleep several times a night. Most midlife women say they can *get to* sleep very easily but have a problem staying asleep. Because we move naturally in and out of REM and non-REM sleep, as long as you go back to sleep soon after waking you may not be losing too many hours of quality sleep. If, however, you take an hour or more trying to get back to sleep each time you wake, you will be losing quality sleep. If this is longstanding, it can lead to sleep anxiety and poor sleep habits, both of which can compound the initial problem.

Whether you have trouble falling asleep or staying asleep, there is rarely a single cause of sleep disturbance in midlife women. Before explaining the role of hormone therapy in this section, I will address some strategies that you can implement on your own that involve reducing some of the sleep-spoiling factors in your environment and inside your body. It is worth mentioning that many healthcare providers, especially medical doctors, often jump straight to sleeping pills for sleep problems. This is because we doctors lack specific training in the management of sleep disorders, but we also often lack the time to carefully define our patients' sleep problems. Most healthcare providers also know about and recommend cognitive behavioral therapy (CBT) for insomnia,[441] and while this has been proven to help in the general population, I find it is only effective in midlife women if used in combination with physical body strategies. So, if you are keen to try a non-medication approach, it is worthwhile being informed about the things you can try yourself before consulting a healthcare provider about a sleep problem.

Strategies to help get to sleep and stay asleep

Difficulty falling asleep is common if you are anxious and many women in this predicament will complain of feeling 'wired and tired'. They feel tired because of the lack of quality sleep but at the same time, feel unable to settle. In these circumstances, levels of the stress hormone called cortisol are likely to be higher than they should be, particularly in the evenings and/or overnight (when they should be very low). Sequential salivary or urine cortisol testing including salivary cortisol awakening response tests can help you determine whether you have high cortisol levels adversely affecting your sleep. If you think you are wired and tired, focus on the de-stressing aspects of the Basic Program and the before-bed sleep strategies listed below.

Optimizing sleep is often about your brain and body's circadian rhythm. There are now informative books available, including one by Dr. Sachin Panda (*The Circadian Code*) to help you understand your body's circadian rhythm and how it relates to good quality sleep and healthy bodily functions. It is important to utilize sunlight to help regulate it, and to monitor and reduce 'artificial blue light' which can disrupt it, especially in the evenings.[442] Accordingly, it is beneficial to get to sleep around the same time every night (before 10 pm if possible) and to reduce the triggers that may wake you up through the night, like sudden noises, bright light, or extreme hot and cold conditions. Having the room at 21°C (about 70°F) or even slightly cooler is ideal, but it probably depends on what temperature you are acclimatized to.

Alcohol and caffeine can both dramatically reduce sleep quality, so it is important to avoid drinking caffeine after 11 am and avoid drinking alcohol 3-4 hours prior to sleep. Preparing for good quality sleep is also a lot about relaxing for 1-2 hours prior to bedtime and reducing stress-inducing activities like watching 'bad-news', violence or 'bad-vibe' television. You can start preparing for sleep as soon as the sun goes down by blocking out bright light, particularly blue light from phones and computers.

Before-bed strategies to improve sleep:

- dim the lights in the house when the sun goes down
- finish eating at least three hours before sleep
- avoid drinking >1-2 alcoholic drinks in the evening
- use blue light blockers for any computer/phone work after dark
- avoid study or computer work in bed
- aim to have your bedroom be as dark as possible
- aim to go to sleep at or before 10 pm
- on rising, aim to get the morning light on your face for 5-10 mins.

Does your gut wake you up?

If being wired and tired does not seem to be your issue, your night-time waking may be a gut problem. The most common gut issue that I have found interferes with sleep is poor digestion. Some of the indicators of poor digestion include reflux or bloating sensations, excess belching, or varying degrees of nausea. These may occur as soon as you try to go to sleep or they may wake you through the night. This is where I advise women to follow the steps to improve digestion (Basic Program) and if needed, to take 'digestive' supplements to strengthen the digestion of their evening meal. Digestive supplements contain 'enzymes' or bitter herbs that help breakdown carbohydrates, proteins and fats. Improving digestion can not only improve sleep, but also help reduce inflammation.

Is pain waking you up?

If you have severe pain, consult your healthcare provider about the causes and get treated. If your sleep is disturbed by mild pain or discomfort, consider a mild analgesic like paracetamol or acetaminophen. Paracetamol/acetaminophen (para-acetylaminophenol) is an over-the-counter medication that is available in most countries. Where it is available, you could try using 500-1000 mg before bed or when you wake in the middle of the night. It has not been studied with respect to sleep, but it is a well-established medication that helps reduce pain and discomfort. I have found many patients say that 500-1000 mg before bed greatly reduces restlessness and improves their sleep quality. Instead of taking it before bed, you could also try taking it when you wake in the middle of the night and feel agitated, worried or restless. Many patients report that it helps them get back to sleep and stay asleep.

It is not uncommon for chronic joint or back pain to be treated with 1000 mg paracetamol 3-4 times a day, so the single nighttime dose I am suggesting is several fold lower than an accepted daily dose.[443] When high doses are taken over long periods of time, paracetamol can be toxic to the liver. It has a notoriously toxic phase I metabolite that, if not cleared quickly in phase II (page 135), may cause liver cell damage.[444] The breakdown of paracetamol requires plenty of detoxification 'resources' in the liver, especially phase II detoxification. To assist in its liver detoxification, I often recommend 1000 mg of the amino acid glycine and/or 500 mg N-acetyl cysteine be taken before bed.

Are your restless legs waking you?

Restless legs or RLS is a well-recognized condition that is not necessarily more common in midlife women and may affect up to 10% of the population.[445] If not addressed, it will tend to worsen during and after midlife. If you have RLS, you will feel an irresistible urge to move your legs especially when resting and when trying to get to sleep.[446] Once you move your legs around, you feel temporary relief of the urge to move, but the relief only lasts 10-20 seconds. It can prevent you getting to sleep and can sometimes wake you from sleep, especially if there are also uncomfortable sensations or pain. If you think you may have RLS, see your healthcare provider to investigate some of the reversible underlying causes like iron deficiency, magnesium or other mineral deficiencies, or small nerve-fiber neuropathy. It is also common in people with advanced kidney disease, in those who consume excess alcohol, and with some medications including anti-nausea, anti-psychotic, antihistamine and anti-depressant medications.

Sleep medications

Sometimes, life circumstances get 'beyond us' and we need help to sleep using a medication. If this is you, consult your healthcare provider about using sleeping tablets, but reserve them for occasional use, being mindful about not becoming a habitual user. Be aware that most sleep medications are habit-forming and are not health-promoting in any way. While sleeping pills can often make you feel like you are sleeping, studies suggest they may not improve your restorative deep sleep. On the contrary, they may cause a reduction in the *quality* of both REM sleep and deep sleep.[447] Moreover, none of 34 studies on sleep medication revealed any benefit in terms of prolonging life or improving health outcomes. In fact, use of sleep medication has been found to be linked to excess mortality, depression, infection, poor driving, poor respiration, and possibly cancer.[448] Similar findings have been found in another large analysis of more than 2.3 million patients using sleep or anti-anxiety medication.[449]

Supplements to help improve sleep

I find the response to supplements somewhat variable between women and better in those who are also following the Basic Program. In general, my favorite tips for midlife women are melatonin, magnesium, the amino acid called glycine, kava, and if there is significant anxiety, ashwagandha.

Melatonin

Melatonin is a hormone that is naturally produced in the body by the pineal gland. Melatonin supplementation is generally well tolerated with no serious short-term or long-term adverse effects in adults.[450] In addition, it isn't associated with dependence, addiction or withdrawal problems. Melatonin has been shown to synchronize circadian rhythms, and improve the onset, duration, and quality of sleep.[451] It also has other benefits including anti-oxidation, anti-inflammation and nerve cell (neuron) longevity.[452] Nevertheless, not everyone benefits from melatonin, so I recommend a trial of an immediate-acting melatonin preparation in addition to the Basic Program and meditation.

Because of melatonin's excellent safety profile, I start with 2-3 mg taken about 30 min before bed. Some women, however, don't notice an effect until they increase this to around 10 mg. I suggest an immediate-release formulation in preference to the slow-release formulations, especially if women feel any kind of 'grogginess' in the mornings. However, some women benefit in terms of night-time waking from a combination of the immediate-release and slow-release formulations and don't suffer from any morning 'grogginess'. Studies are underway on the efficacy and benefits of higher doses (up to 100 mg) in reducing oxidative stress in the brain and in improving cancer therapy outcomes.[453]

Glycine

Glycine is a sweet-tasting amino acid found in protein-rich food such as meat, fish, dairy products, cheese, and vegetables. Studies have shown that glycine can promote a deeper level of sleep, especially REM sleep,[454] and reduce night-time body temperature,[455] which is probably why it works well in midlife women. I have found this amino acid to be very helpful in midlife women for both falling asleep and staying asleep and this is consistent with the few clinical studies available.[456] It is extremely safe with usual oral doses being 2000-3000 mg taken just before sleep.

In addition to promoting sleep, glycine has liver-protecting properties similar to N-acetyl cysteine or NAC, a compound used to protect the liver after paracetamol overdose.[457] In fact, glycine also promotes bile formation, hemoglobin synthesis (red blood cells), and helps protect the gut wall.[458] I also recommend 1000-2000 mg glycine taken after meals to help reduce sugar cravings. Its beneficial effect probably has something to do with the fact that it is a 'sweet' amino acid, but it has no ill-effects on blood sugar or blood insulin levels.

Magnesium and taurine

When taken before bed, magnesium can reduce night-time muscle cramps and/or soreness and can promote relaxation if sleep is disturbed by stress or anxiety.[459] Although not everyone feels the benefit with regards to sleep, because magnesium deficiency is common, I often prescribe between 250 and 1000 mg of either magnesium-citrate, magnesium-chelate or magnesium-L-threonate before bed. When there is excess stress and anxiety, I add in about 500 mg of the amino acid taurine. Taurine has been shown to have sleep-promoting, anti-neuroinflammation and neuro-protective properties. It can also increase the amount of circulating relaxation-promoting compounds called GABA and reduce the amount of circulating levels of the stress hormone cortisol.[460] Other supplements that I recommend less commonly but which are more often taken by women on their own accord include tryptophan, chamomile, kava, and valerian.

Bedtime therapies to help promote sleep at-a-glance:
- 500-1000 mg paracetamol
- 500 mg N-acetyl-cysteine (especially if taking paracetamol)
- 2-10 mg melatonin
- 1000-3000 mg glycine
- 400-800 mg magnesium citrate, chelate or L-threonate
- herbal tea lemon balm, passionflower, chamomile.

Hormone therapy for sleep according to Zone
Zone 1 and Zone 2
Night-time waking can be reduced by taking oral (micronized) progesterone before bed. Progesterone seems to improve the ability of your body to relax at night via a reduction of sympathetic nervous system output. Oral progesterone is known to be converted to compounds in the body that stimulate GABA activity, and thus relaxation.[461] If anxiety and difficulty falling asleep remain a problem despite taking oral progesterone, you may benefit from an increased dose and if that is not an option, a trial of 2.5-5% progesterone cream applied to the back of the neck before bed (except during cycle days 1-10). See your healthcare provider for these options.

Zone 3 and Zone 4
Oral progesterone can also greatly reduce your night-time waking in Zone 3 and Zone 4.[461] If you also have low estrogen symptoms, such as hot flushing

and vaginal dryness and you have no contraindications to estrogen, you should ask your healthcare provider about adding transdermal estrogen. If you need to use estrogen-containing hormone therapy for extended periods, I recommend the Estrogen Clearing Program to help you clear the estrogens and to help reduce the long-term cancer-promoting effects of the estrogen.

Brain health

Midlife is a great time to start thinking about protecting your brain and reducing your chances of suffering from debilitating cognitive decline and dementia. There are many factors that can increase risk of dementia, and no two people will get it for the same reasons. It is not just about your genetics and, as the research into this devastating disease grows, we are understanding more about the factors that make us more susceptible.[90] The more we know about the disease, the more complex it seems to be. Its complexity is the reason why nearly all 1,000 or so dementia drug trials have made little to no difference in its progression.[89] As a result, research is now moving towards uncovering the factors that contribute to getting dementia. In this way, the research can help us devise ways to *prevent*, rather than treat dementia. In fact, clinicians and researchers are now using a multi-directional preventative approach using lifestyle, diet, and exercise.[91]

Sufficient quality sleep is key to brain health

Getting enough good quality sleep is now considered key to being and staying healthy throughout your lifetime. Longstanding poor sleep increases the risk of developing many chronic diseases including diabetes (increases dementia risk by at least 2-fold), heart disease and depression.[462] As we get older, for some reason, we lose time in deep sleep, yet this is the most important time when our brains undergo synchronized brainwaves that help 'clean out' toxic waste products through the activity of what are known as the glymphatics (**page 53**).

If you have a sleep partner, be sure to ask them if you snore, and if you do, regardless of whether they think you stop breathing during sleep or not, get a sleep study done. Sleep hypopnea/apnea can cause you to 'wake' throughout the night, even if you don't remember and it can greatly reduce your restorative deep sleep. Having day-time sleepiness is an indicator of sleep apnea, so take note of this if you have it.[75]

Most of us who feel we don't sleep well experience either being easily disturbed, waking multiple times through the night or feeling unrefreshed in the morning. Whatever your sleep issue is, sleep tracking devices can be very useful in showing you the nature of your sleep disturbance. According to a recent study, a sleep tracking ring is 50-60% accurate at determining the three levels of sleep, light sleep, deep sleep or non-REM and REM sleep.[463] One study in 20 women showed that just wearing a sleep tracker and doing a sleep journal improved sleep quality and reduced sleep disturbance.[464] In my personal and clinical experience with sleep trackers, tracking sleep parameters encourages a healthy awareness of the diet/lifestyle factors that influence quality of sleep. Even though the sleep tracker technology isn't 100% accurate in differentiating between light, non-REM, and REM sleep, sleep trackers can help motivate people to engage in activities that improve sleep and reduce the ones that worsen it. I find the tracking rings are easier to wear than the wrist bands or other devices.

Menopausal hormone therapy for the brain – what the research tells us
Menopausal hormone therapy (MHT) is covered in detail from **page 231** onwards. If you have night-time hot flushes (night sweats), menopausal hormone therapy (MHT) can help reduce the frequency of the nighttime waking (with flushing) and night sweats.[74] It follows that when you improve your sleep, you improve your brain health. The studies examining a link between MHT and improving brain health, however, have not been conclusive. Studies on the factors that increase the risk of dementia are notoriously challenging to stage and to interpret. For example, different conclusions were obtained from two studies of hundreds of thousands of menopausal women in Finland. The first study, published in 2017 found that using MHT for 10 years or more was linked to a *lower* risk of dementia, but the second published

in 2019 found that any use, including long term use, of MHT was linked to a slightly *higher* risk of dementia.[465] These conflicting study outcomes result from trying to get meaningful information from large population studies that have large volumes of data which are incomplete or missing.

Several other population and interventional studies have been published, but unfortunately, they have not been able to clarify the relationship between MHT and dementia with some demonstrating a reduced risk[466] (estrogen only MHT), an increased [467] risk (only with combined estrogen and progestin) or a neutral effect.[468] One study found that late-onset menopause and MHT both had a positive effect on the *volume* of the memory area of the brain[469] while another showed that regardless of MHT, menopausal women with the lowest cholesterol levels were at *highest* risk.[468] A study of more than 1.3 million South Korean menopausal women found that tibolone and *oral* estrogen MHT were linked to a higher risk of dementia, whereas transdermal estrogen with or without a progestogen was not (explained on **page 232**).[470] It does appear more certain that women who arrive at menopause before the age of 40 and don't take MHT, are at a higher risk of getting dementia. This is especially the case if they had surgery or chemotherapy to remove their ovaries.[471, 472]

Experts from the Mayo Clinic have stated that:

The relation of hormone therapy with the risk of dementia is complex. Hormone therapy may have beneficial, neutral, or harmful effects on the brain. Hormone therapy should be guided by the clinical characteristics of the women being treated.[473]

Experts from the National Institutes of Health say:

Among senior women, the implications of menopausal hormone therapy use beyond age 65 years vary by types, routes, and strengths. In general, risk reductions appear to be greater with low rather than medium or high doses, vaginal or transdermal rather than oral preparations, and with E2 rather than conjugated (equine) estrogen.[466]

High blood pressure

One of the most important indicators of poor blood-vessel health is high blood pressure. Having high blood pressure increases the risk of having a poor blood supply to the brain and can worsen all the other factors that contribute to dementia.[474] In people at risk for dementia, using medication to optimize blood pressure is linked to a better outcome.[475] High blood pressure results from a dysfunction in the cells that line the inside of blood vessels called endothelial cells. High blood pressure follows 'endothelial dysfunction', and endothelial dysfunction has numerous underlying contributors including inflammation.[476] Without going into the subject of blood pressure too far, reducing your whole-body inflammation via the Basic Program will help you maintain healthy endothelial function, a healthy blood pressure and in turn, a healthy brain.[477]

Blood sugar

If the thought of having diabetes doesn't help you resolve a sugar addiction, maybe the thought of getting dementia does. Having diabetes, particularly poorly controlled diabetes, increases your risk of dementia through several mechanisms including blood vessel dysfunction, inflammation, and changes in metabolism.[478] Even having pre-diabetes with occasional high blood sugar and a high insulin level may predispose to cognitive decline.[479] Following the Basic Program, especially the anti-inflammatory diet, is the perfect plan to reverse and avoid pre-diabetes and can go a long way in reversing diabetes in most people. One study has been able to show that the Mediterranean diet can reduce diabetes and in turn, reduce risk of dementia.[91]

Brain insults to be aware of:

- head injuries including concussion and amnesia
- heavy metals including mercury, lead, aluminum
- inflamogens including mycotoxins from mold
- chronic or hidden sinus, jaw or dental infections.

Head injuries

Not many midlife women have occupations or hobbies that predispose them to head injuries but take note if you are a keen soccer player, boxer, or player of any kind of contact sport. Single significant or multiple small knocks to the head can in some people be a disaster later in life.[480] If you *do* get a knock on the head, make sure you keep yourself in a quiet place with dim lights and very little sound for the time you are recovering and if you are not taking blood thinning medication, take a generous dose of omega-3 oils to help reduce inflammation.[481]

Heavy metal toxicity

Mercury, lead and aluminum can be directly toxic to nerves and the brain. Theoretically, at least, our lifetime exposure to these heavy metals via a toxic polluted environment could be proportional to our risk of dementia.[482] It doesn't make sense to me that mercury, a known neurotoxin, has been used as the most common dental caries filler for more than 80 years. Amalgam fillings are linked to having mercury in the brain[483] and other organs.[484] Sweden and Norway have already banned amalgam fillings, while Ireland, Finland, and Slovakia are planning to ban them over the next few years for 'neurological' reasons. Meanwhile, I suggest that my patients investigate alternative restoration dental fillers and to consult a biological dentist if they have amalgams that they'd like removed. While data showing a link between amalgam use and dementia may take years, it is never too late to make decisions about your health that could make a difference.

You should also be aware of how to avoid mercury in food. At least one study has found that the amount of brain mercury is linked to the number of seafood meals consumed.[485] For this reason, avoid eating large deep-sea varieties of fish, and favor small varieties including anchovies, sardines, and mackerel.

Mycotoxins are inflammatory and can affect the brain

I first covered this topic on **pages 77 & 190**. Those of us who treat patients with mold-related illness can see that inhaled mycotoxins can lead to body and brain inflammatory symptoms, including headaches, brain fog and cognitive issues. Little is known about the extent or nature of brain inflammation that occurs,[169] but it is possible that longstanding mycotoxin-related whole-body and brain inflammation can lead to early cognitive decline and dementia. However, not everyone gets noticeably unwell from breathing in excessive mycotoxins.[486] Theoretically, if you have more hormones to process in your body at midlife, it is possible that you may be more susceptible to symptoms of toxic overload because exposure to excess mycotoxins can lead to an increase in your body's overall toxic burden.

If you suspect you may have some mold-related symptoms, take note of musty smells in your house and investigate any water intrusions that may have occurred through a leaky roof or wall, a burst pipe, or a leaky fridge (with ice-maker), dishwasher or air conditioner. If you do find water intrusions, instead of just repairing the intrusions, get a moldy building specialist to determine the full extent of water damage that needs addressing.

Chronic infections in the sinus cavities and jaw

Poor oral health (gingivitis, dental caries, tooth loss, tooth abscess) appears to be linked to an increased risk of developing cognitive impairment and dementia.[487] Does this mean poor oral health can cause dementia? No, it is too early to tell from the limited study findings we have so far. If you are concerned about your oral health or concerned about getting dementia, be sure to ask your dentist to organize X-rays and/or a cone CT of your jaw. A CT is perhaps better because you want to check that you don't have any silent chronic bone sepsis or infection, a tooth abscess, or both.[488]

Chronic or recurrent sinusitis may also be linked to dementia but, again, we don't know whether this is a cause-and-effect relationship.[489] We also don't know whether it is the infection (usually a bacteria) or the associated inflammation that may be the problem. What can you do about it? If you have a lot of sinus issues, try regular sinus rinsing with warm saline water. You can add a small amount of xylitol to the saline to help break down the coating of mucus (biofilm) that could be hiding and protecting the bacteria and mold. You may also want to use a small amount of probiotic (e.g., lactobacillus) solution dabbed, not sprayed, into the nose to help encourage the growth of normal flora in your nose and then sinus cavities. In severe and chronic forms of sinusitis, thorough sinus rinsing by an ear-nose-throat surgeon using specialized equipment may be warranted.

Reducing your risk of dementia at-a-glance:

- focus on improving your sleep if it is disturbed
- focus on getting quality REM and non-REM sleep
- eliminate or treat any sleep apnea
- avoiding use of sleeping pills on a regular basis
- check your blood pressure regularly and ensure it is optimal
- check your blood glucose levels are optimal
- wear head protective gear where head injury is a risk
- have your dentist exclude chronic dental sepsis (abscesses)
- ask your healthcare provider about progesterone and/or estrogen hormone therapy.

Heart health

Cardiovascular disease remains the leading cause of death in women, but only around 45% of women polled in the USA are aware of this or the fact that their risk can accelerate at midlife, and around the time of menopause.[490] Women are more likely to perceive that their weight or breast cancer are the major dangers. Being overweight or obese increases the risk of breast cancer, cardiovascular disease and death.[491] Although the research data is an absolute minefield to make sense of, some experts agree that starting MHT at or early after Zone 4 is beneficial in terms of cardiovascular health, in addition to lowering rates of diabetes, reducing insulin resistance, and protecting from bone loss.[492] However to date, there are no formal recommendations to prescribe menopausal hormone therapy for the purpose of preventing cardiovascular disease. It is best to explore all other risk-reducing strategies to improve your long-term cardiovascular health.

The Australian Heart Foundation and American Heart Association outline some of the ways to reduce your risk of heart disease.

Heart disease risk-reducing tips:

- stop smoking
- monitor your BP so it is maintained at or below 130/80
- lose weight if your body mass index is 26 or greater
- exercise for a total of 2-3 hours a week (in 3-4 workouts)
- attend to any risks for diabetes
- reduce alcohol to 1-2 glasses 2-3 times a week
- manage any chronic inflammatory conditions
- avoid eating trans-fats, packaged/snack foods, fast foods
- reduce processed meats like deli-style, cured, smoked cuts.

Your heart and red meat

Many heart disease studies to date have shown a link between red meat consumption and an increased risk of heart disease. But does this mean that *all* red meat is unhealthy for your heart? I would say, no. In fact, there are important and relevant differences between fresh unprocessed red meat from grass-fed cattle and red meat products from industrial-grain-fed cattle. In addition, perhaps the *way* the meat is cooked also influences whether it is good or bad for your heart. I discussed some of this information on red meat and cooking methods on **pages 118-120** when explaining the anti-inflammatory diet. Briefly, red meat from grass-fed cattle has significantly higher concentrations of heart healthy omega-3 fatty acids than grain-fed cattle.[493] In fact, the omega-3 levels are comparable to Australian wild-caught fish.[494] Moreover, red meat, including meat from sheep, has higher concentrations of another heart healthy fat called docosapentaenoic acid (DPA) and we already know that DPA-rich foods are equally if not more beneficial than either EPA or DHA (omega-3 fatty acids) in reducing risk of heart disease.[495, 496]

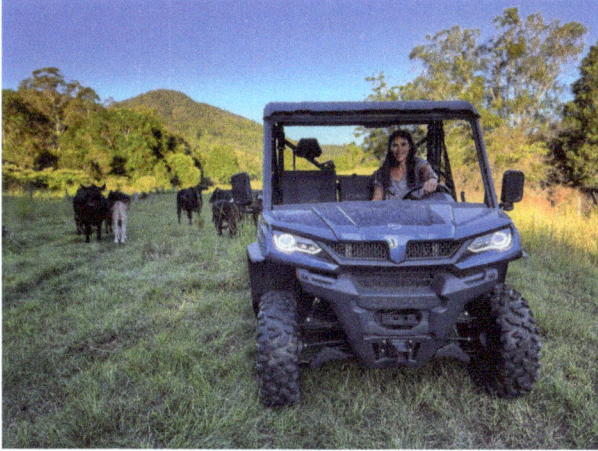

Raising our own grass-fed beef using rotational grazing and regenerative farming principles

The other problem with industrially raised beef

Industrial beef is from cattle that are fattened up or 'finished' in an industrial feedlot before slaughter. In the USA, cattle are nearly all raised and fed in a feedlot. In Australia, most animals are grass fed, but 'finished' in a feedlot prior to slaughter. Feedlot food consists initially of hay, which is then changed progressively to a diet of about 85% grain (mostly corn and smaller amounts of oats, barley, and sorghum) and 15% additives. The additives are numerous and include extra nutrients, 'growth promoters' and chemicals to reduce the 'acidosis' that the cattle get from eating grain that isn't a natural food for them. Most feedlots also include antibiotics which are said to be 'safe'. Apart from the food that cattle eat, it is worth being mindful of the poor conditions that these animals live in. If you have ever been to a feedlot, the smell can literally knock you over. The cattle are confined to small yards where they cannot do anything except stand around between meals in their foul-smelling 'manure mud'. They exist like this day after day, with nowhere to walk, no shade and nowhere clean or dry to sit.

When you raise your own cattle, like I do, you can very much appreciate how cattle love to walk and run around a paddock and prefer to rest with each other in the shade. We practice holistic farming where we graze smaller paddocks on rotation. It's uncanny, but my cattle will let me know when they have 'finished' a paddock. What I mean by this is, when they have run out of clean, unsoiled (by their excrement) grass, they let me know by standing at the gate and either staring me down or bellowing. In my opinion, holding cattle in a feedlot is not only inhumane, but also produces lower-quality meat. The feedlot industry, however, is about economics, not about looking after the cattle and certainly not about the health of the product. Given research has shown vast differences between meat from cattle finished in feed-lots and meat from cattle raised entirely in grassy paddocks, perhaps future Heart Foundation recommendations will include grass-fed meat choices.

Cattle and the future of our planet

If you do care about the environment, perhaps you would consider caring about cattle and, for that matter, all grass-eating ruminants. Contrary to some views that would have cows and ruminants abolished altogether (because of their methane-containing flatulence), many farmers around the world are starting to realize the critical role that ruminant animals like cattle play in *nurturing* our planet. Where there are no cattle, there is no manure, and where there is no manure, there are no healthy microbiome-rich soils. This means no nutrition-rich vegetables/grains. In fact, many people in the agricultural industry are realizing that eliminating the cattle industry would be an absolute disaster for the environment. It is clear that ruminant animals do a fantastic job of regenerating our soils. For them to do this, however, they need to be managed in a particular way consistent with regenerative farming practices.[497] If you are interested in reading more about this, I recommend a fascinating book called *Call of the Reed Warbler* about an Australian farmer and his journey from industrial to regenerative farming.

By supporting your local grass-fed meat producers, especially those involved in regenerative farming practices, you can raise awareness of this important farming practice, and at the same time, enjoy the health benefits of grass-fed and finished beef/lamb/poultry/pork, as well as contribute to regeneration of our soils and the planet.

Back to the heart of women

Before menopause, women enjoy a lower heart disease risk than men. After menopause, that risk unfortunately increases and, over a few short years, reaches a risk level that equals men. Even so, women can still get heart disease in midlife before menopause, especially if there is a strong family history of heart attacks at an early age. The ethnic groups most at risk for heart problems before or after menopause include South Asians, Africans, African Caribbeans, indigenous North and South Americans, indigenous Australians, and Pacific Islanders including the Māori.[498, 499]

Tips to help reduce heart disease risk in any Zone:

- eat unprocessed fresh foods
- avoid processed sugary or packaged food
- exercise regularly and make it fun
- focus on losing weight if you need to
- ensure optimal sleep
- if you have night sweats, ask for treatment
- if you have hot flushes, ask for treatment
- ask yourself if you need a major health check up
- make sure your blood pressure is optimal
- never ignore chest pain, and get checked
- reduce stress
- go dancing, watch a light comedy, laugh
- go bushwalking or just get out and enjoy nature
- try doing a gratitude diary
- nurture friendships, especially with those who are like-minded, inspirational and high-integrity
- nurture and spend time with your loved ones
- take time to focus on nurturing yourself.

Libido

Low libido

If your libido has tanked or vanished, ask yourself whether you are taking any medications or substances that could be causing or worsening the situation. These include birth control pills, anti-depressants (particularly SSRIs like citalopram, escitalopram, and fluoxetine), codeine-containing analgesics, seizure medications, blood pressure medications like beta blockers and excess alcohol. Also consider whether you are just too tired from poor sleep, have lost confidence in the way you look, or have any unresolved trauma or unfulfilled expectations. Unrewarding sexual experiences can also contribute to a waning desire.

Our health and fitness play an important role, and if you're unfit and don't feel well generally, like many women, you won't feel at all sexy. Vaginal dryness is a common problem after menopause, but it can also occur before menopause. It can prevent both desire and arousal. I review the effective treatments for this on **page 242** that involve restoring healthy function to your vulvo-vaginal mucous membranes.[500]

Hormone therapy for libido

If you are in peak fitness/health and still experiencing low libido, you may want to consider hormone therapy. Although there is only a weak link between low libido and blood hormone levels of estrogen or testosterone, the combination of estrogen and testosterone has been shown to help some women in Zone 4 with low libido,[501] but not women in Zone 1 or Zone 2.[502] If you are in Zone 4 or in Zone 3 with low estrogen symptoms, and you are distressed about your low libido, I suggest seeing a healthcare provider who is experienced in diagnosing hypoactive sexual desire disorder (HSDD) and prescribing hormone therapies including dehydroepiandrosterone (DHEA) and testosterone. Part of your clinical work-up for testosterone therapy will be to exclude other possible causes of your low libido and a blood testosterone level. This testosterone level is not done for the purposes of making a diagnosis, but rather to obtain a baseline upon which to monitor levels in future. So far, the known long-term adverse health consequences of properly prescribed and monitored testosterone therapy are not too disturbing and include minor changes in blood lipids and blood pressure, an increase in acne and an increase in coarse facial hair.[501]

Experienced practitioners who are used to prescribing complex compounded formulations often treat libido with a variety of topical agents that can be put in and around the vagina or administered via a nasal spray. The vaginal preparations include creams containing DHEA[503] and/or low dose naltrexone and oxytocin gel.[504] Medications that can help when given via the intranasal route include PT-141[505, 506] and oxytocin.[507]

Bone health

Bone health is important to every woman. Bone loss after about age 35 is normal, but if you take steps to maintain healthy bones, you can reduce your bone loss at midlife and beyond. Poor bone mass and strength is a major cause of lethal hip and other fractures as we age. Anyone who works in a hospital knows how common fractures are in older women (and men) and how commonly a seemingly simple fracture can lead to catastrophic medical outcomes and death. Bone loss is referred to as osteopenia and, when severe, osteoporosis. Although taking steps to prevent osteoporosis is more effective the earlier you do it, working on healthy bones is an effective strategy starting any time, including at midlife.[213] If you have osteopenia or osteoporosis at the time of menopause, you need to work hard (literally physically hard) to maintain the bone strength you have, let alone improve it. Medications can only marginally, if at all, increase bone density and strength. This is why knowing how to optimize your bone strength from midlife onwards can make a huge difference in later life.

> **Strategies to help maintain strong bones:**
>
> - eat a fresh, low-inflammation diet (Basic Program)
> - ensure adequate calcium and minerals from dietary sources
> - partake in regular weight-bearing or resistance exercise
> - ensure optimal vitamin D levels and supplement if needed
> - consider regularly supplementing with magnesium, vitamin K2, and boron.

Ensuring a healthy-bone lifestyle: The Basic Program

The Basic Program, with its anti-inflammatory strategies, is a great place to start for bone health. Reducing whole-body inflammation helps to maintain healthy bone by optimizing the hormones that keep calcium, important trace elements, and other components of bone in perpetual balance.[508] Excess inflammation interrupts this balance and favors bone breakdown over bone formation.[509] The stress reduction component of the Basic Program is also important for bone health because we know that excessive levels of the stress hormone cortisol are linked to more bone breakdown and less bone-building.[510]

Obesity and bone

Being overweight influences your bone density and strength both negatively and positively. The negative effects are due to the tendency to be sedentary, to have obesity-related inflammation and, in some people, to have faulty ovulation.[511] The positive effects are due to the excess weight applying chronic bone-building stress on the bone, plus, an increased level of the fat tissue-derived estrogen called estrone. If you are overweight or obese (BMI >30) you can promote your bone strength by eating an anti-inflammatory diet and doing the right kinds of exercise, particularly bone-building, weight-bearing and resistance exercise. While being obese can help protect you from bone loss, it may increase your risk of hormone-dependent cancers, especially breast cancer.[216]

A bone-healthy diet

To support bone health through diet, start by eating fresh foods and observing the anti-inflammatory diet part of the Basic Program. Eating calcium-rich foods on a regular basis is also important, examples of calcium-rich foods are chia seeds (soaked chia seeds are also a great source of fiber), nuts, cheese, sardines, pulses (make sure you soak these well before pressure-cooking them), almonds, dark leafy greens, rhubarb, amaranth, tofu, and figs (watch the sugar content). I advise women to consume non-dairy calcium-rich foods in preference to cow's milk. If you want to consume cow's milk products, I suggest favoring organic versions and avoiding large amounts of milk (more than a 'dash' in coffee/tea). Remember that industrially-raised and managed animals (includes many dairy cows in most countries) are exposed to all manner of xeno-estrogens which increases the likelihood that we are exposed to them in their milk produce. Soy milk is an alternative to cow's milk but, again, I advise consuming organic versions to reduce your exposure to pesticides and other xeno-estrogens. It's also worth noting that many people who are sensitive to dairy are also sensitive to soy products.

While soy and soy-based foods contain large amounts of health-promoting phytoestrogens, drinking soy hasn't been found to be particularly beneficial for menopausal bones or symptoms.[512] Other nut milks like almond, cashew, and macadamia milk have some advantages over cow's milk in that they contain as much, if not more, calcium than cow's milk and contain significantly less carbohydrate. For example, one cup of 2% fat cow's milk contains approximately 120 calories, 5 g of fat, 8 g of protein, and 12 g of carbohydrates. One cup of almond (or macadamia) milk contains 35 (or 25) calories, 2.5 (or 2) g of fat, 1 (or <1) g of protein, and 1 g of carbohydrate. Milks made with hazelnuts or walnuts tend to be higher in fat and higher in calories. Again, I would advise choosing organic versions of all nut milks where possible to reduce your exposure to pesticides and other xeno-estrogens.

Exercise to prevent bone loss

Combining impact exercise with resistance training seems to be the best choice in terms of preserving or improving bone density in pre-menopausal and post-menopausal women.[513] Neither whole-body vibration techniques or walking/jogging have been shown yet to significantly increase bone density, but both have muscle and agility benefits that could offset the risks of low bone density.[514] Traditional progressive resistance training has been shown to help increase bone density, with improvements in bone mass, muscle mass, and muscle size and strength. Your weight training does not need to be particularly strenuous and should not be stressful to perform. Most of the research data points to moderate exercise rather than high-intensity exercise and this is likely because high-intensity exercise can increase your stress hormone (cortisol) levels. If you do want to participate in intense exercise on a regular basis, you should limit the length and number of sessions per week. Doing it frequently and for lengthy periods can increase the risk of fatigue, injury, and an increased stress response.

If you are trying to lose weight, high-intensity exercise can sometimes slow weight loss due to the body's response to the stress. The increased stress can increase your cortisol levels, and this can reduce your muscle mass, thus reducing the 'power batteries' that drive your fat-burning ability.[515] Depending on how long and high your cortisol levels are elevated, cortisol can also increase body fat, especially around your midriff, even if you are eating less than 500 calories a day. If you are serious about losing weight, I would recommend a program that aims to strengthen and build muscle, and this may mean getting an assessment by an experienced exercise physiologist to work out a program uniquely suited to your body type and your preferences. I also recommend taking protein drinks containing 30-40 g protein (with high-leucine content, like collagen or whey protein) immediately after your workouts. This along with supplementing your vitamin D and other micronutrients has been found to be helpful in muscle building and maintenance and in weight loss programs.[516]

Another form of exercise that is not immediately obvious as a bone-benefiting exercise is tai chi. Tai chi has been shown to help preserve bone in menopausal women, and it can also improve body pain, improve general health, vitality and mental health.[517] When you consider the muscle work that is involved in holding the positions during the slow tai chi movements, you can understand how it can have such positive effects on bone health.

The maintenance of exercise that includes muscle-building exercise is critical in avoiding the muscle loss that occurs with age. Age-related muscle loss is called 'sarcopenia' (*sarco* = muscle; *penia* = shrink/reduce).[518] Here is what the authors of a European consensus said in their 2018 revised paper:

In terms of human health, sarcopenia increases risk of falls and fractures; impairs ability to perform activities of daily living; is associated with cardiac disease, respiratory disease and cognitive impairment; leads to mobility disorders; and contributes to lowered quality of life, loss of independence or need for long-term care placement, and death.[519]

Many women and men notice a reduced ability to build muscle as they age. This is likely due to a drop in the body's natural 'anabolic' or muscle-building hormones, like human growth hormone. It is important not to try to counter-act this loss by increasing the intensity and frequency of workouts. This can increase cortisol levels, which can end up doing the opposite, and causing muscle loss. It is better to become smarter about how, when, and what sort of exercise you do. I make my muscle-building workouts easy and accessible, using bands,[520] a bar and wearing blood flow restriction cuffs.[521] I do these 20-30-minute workouts in my own home at least five times a week depending on how much outdoor physical activity I am doing on my property. To complete the workout, I take a small protein meal or smoothie with 30-50 g protein.

Blood flow restriction cuffs are somewhat 'high tech' and take a bit of getting used to because they can be quite uncomfortable to use at first. The bands work by distending or stretching the veins in your limbs, which triggers the release of your own body's 'trophic' (muscle building) hormones. The use of blood flow restriction during exercise may sound weird to many, but it is an ingenious technique that was first discovered in Japan due to its effectiveness in accelerating recovery rate after injury or stroke.[521] The first therapeutic studies were performed in older people with the aim of helping to improve their rehabilitation process and get them functioning independently more rapidly. These days the cuffs are used by all ages to help build muscle.[522, 523] There are no studies yet on this technique and building bone, but by building stronger muscles and increasing the body's own trophic hormone, they are an excellent support for any bone-building program that you do.

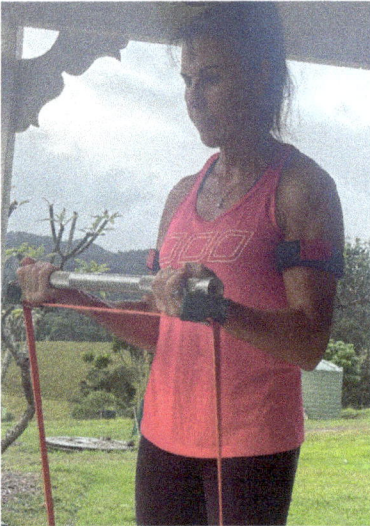

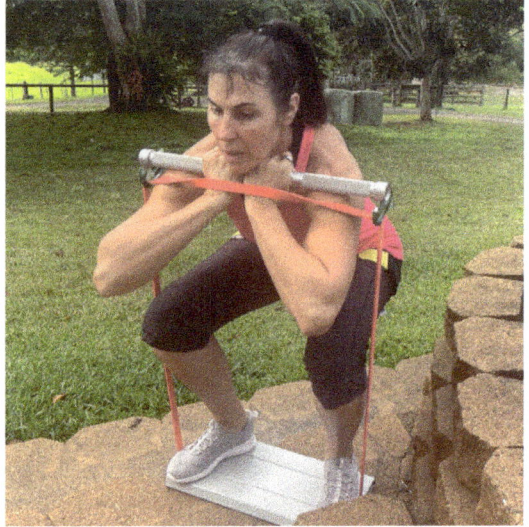

Doing some basic strength exercises in the fresh air and with restriction bands

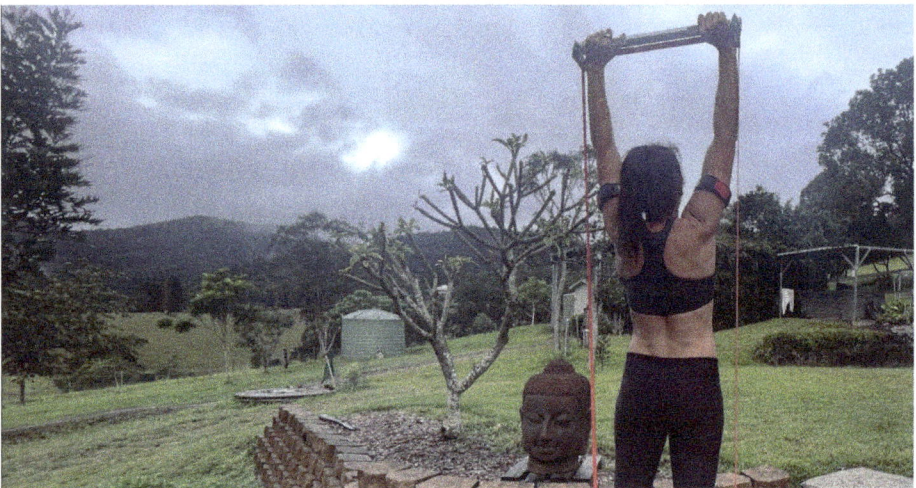

Reaching for the sky in the shoulder press to build a strong back and shoulders

Supplements used to help support bone health

Bone is a very dynamic body tissue that perpetually responds to alterations in your diet and nutritional status. Your bone is constantly undergoing turnover by bone-osteoclasts (breaking bone down) and bone-osteoblasts (building bone up). When these two bone cells are working in balance, they constantly remodel bone while balancing the collagen and mineral content to maintain bone strength. Bones are made up of about 35% protein (mostly collagen protein) and about 65% trace minerals, like calcium, phosphate, magnesium, phosphorous, potassium, boron, copper, iron, zinc, selenium, molybdenum, and others. Sometimes supplementing a healthy diet with these minerals may be useful in supporting bone maintenance and building.

Calcium

Most women get enough calcium from eating calcium-rich foods on a regular basis. In fact, taking supplemental calcium should be directed by your health-care professional, because taking 500 mg or more of calcium in supplement form has been linked to heart disease.[524] Having said that, you are probably safe to take up to 250 mg a day in supplemental form without getting an assessment, but take it with around 80-160 μg vitamin K2 daily to offset calcium deposition in the arteries.[525] Also, if you are taking both vitamin D and calcium supplements, have your blood vitamin D and calcium levels checked periodically. Other vital supplements for bone health include a daily dose of at least 600 mg magnesium and 3-6 mg boron.[526] I reserve prescribing calcium supplementation for women who have suboptimal bone density and have low-normal or low blood levels of calcium even after their vitamin D levels have been optimized and vitamin K2 has been added.

Vitamin D, the multi-talented hormone

Vitamin D should really be referred to as *Hormone D* because its structure and function matches that of a hormone, not a 'vitamin'. It has numerous key roles in the body, but one of its important roles is in the regulation of calcium levels in the body, particularly in the blood and bone. Our own bodies can manufacture vitamin D through a series of steps in the gut, kidney, liver, and finally, in the skin. The synthesis of the 'active' form of vitamin D (called *1alpha,25-dihydrocholecalciferol* or *1,25[OH]-D3* or *simply Vitamin D3*) in our skin is dependent on the UV light contained within natural sunlight.

The production of vitamin D in your skin is reduced:

- in winter compared to summer
- if you have a dark (especially black) complexion
- after the age of 65
- with the use of any sunscreen and is fully blocked if using 15+ or higher protection-factor
- if you have inadequate intake or absorption of nutrients (poor gut health)
- in severe kidney disease or other chronic illness.

Vitamin D also plays an important role in blood sugar control (and preventing diabetes), immune function, reducing levels of inflammation, regulating mood and emotions, reducing the risk of autoimmunity, managing oxidative stress, and protecting/regenerating nerves.[527] It is one amazing hormone! You can get vitamin D from foods like cod liver oil, sardines, mushrooms, egg yolks, and vitamin-D-fortified foods.

Some women only need to supplement vitamin D during the winter months because they can maintain healthy levels through diet and sun exposure during warmer months. If you have a history of low vitamin D, an autoimmune disorder, a neurological disorder, pre-diabetes, or diabetes, you may need supplementing all year round so talk to your healthcare provider about the dose that would suit you and to arrange annual or more frequent vitamin D (and calcium) level checks.

Vitamin K2

Vitamin K2 is a recently discovered 'hormone-like vitamin' also known as menaquinone-7. It has been shown to improve bone density in the lumbar spine in menopausal women and, in experimental mice, it has been shown to reduce calcium deposits within arteries.[528] The laying down of calcium outside the bones and in the arteries, heart valves and other tissues is called 'extra-osseous deposition', and is linked to chronic diseases such as cardio-vascular disease and stroke. Studies are underway that will hopefully tell us if vitamin K2 can reduce the amount of calcium deposited in our arteries.[529, 530] When taking vitamin K2, be aware that it can have some vitamin K1 activity, so if you're taking the blood thinner called warfarin, you need to monitor your bleeding results (INR level).[531]

Boron

Boron is a trace element that plays an important role in animal and human health, particularly bone health, immune function, reproduction, and brain health.[532] Given most of the information so far comes from animal research, there are no established guidelines as to what constitutes boron deficiency in women. Results from early pilot studies suggest boron deficiency may be linked to an increased risk of arthritis, poor bone architecture[526] and poor cognition[533] but these studies have not been repeated.

Boron is abundant in plants grown in boron-rich soil and a diet full of fresh fruits and vegetables from these soils will usually provide a bone-healthy amount of boron. If your fruit and vegetables are, however, grown in boron-deficient soils, you may not be getting a bone-healthy amount of boron in your diet. The average daily boron intake from the diet is around 1-1.5 mg in boron-sufficient areas but may be less than 0.5 mg daily in deficient areas.[526] The fact that boron is the main ingredient in borax, a popular cleaning product, may be part of the reason why many people link the words boron and 'toxic'. Nevertheless, toxicity studies show that boron is barely toxic even at doses 60,000 times higher than is found in a plentiful boron-rich food diet. In an emergency room study, doses up to 88 g (a single 'poison dose') did not lead to any deaths or significant symptoms.[534] Beware though, that if you inhale borax or other types of boron, it can damage your lungs.

In a review of 11 studies in more than 500 women and men, it was found that a daily dose of 3-9 mg may be effective in preventing bone loss and maintaining bone mass.[526] Further long-term studies should be performed, however given many nutritional studies are not funded (because products being studied cannot be patented and monetized), this may be a long time coming. Because of what we know regarding boron's safety profile, I recommend boron for my patients who have issues with weak bones or early arthritis. I often request boron testing (hair and urine) before supplementation commences. The dose is usually between 6-9 mg daily to start with and after 12 months or so, about 3 mg daily for maintenance depending on clinical response. Note that the World Health Organization's acceptable safe range of boron intake is 1-13 mg per day.

If you take a boron supplement, choose one that is made by a reputable supplement company containing boron citrate and/or boron glycinate. Long term supplementation with boron appears to be safe, given the fact that it doesn't accumulate in the body and is readily eliminated via the kidneys. Although I usually suggest a boron-only supplement, for small daily doses of boron, it can be taken as a combined supplement with other important bone trace minerals such as potassium, molybdenum, strontium, silica, zinc, and copper.[535] Women usually have higher copper levels than men because estrogen tends to decrease the elimination of copper and increase the elimination of zinc. For these reasons, I recommend having your blood copper and zinc levels checked before taking supplements of these two. I also recommend measuring thyroid function and urine iodine levels before boron supplementation and on a yearly basis thereafter. In some areas where environmental boron is high, the rate of thyroid goiter has been higher than expected.[536]

Sunlight and sunscreen

Sunlight has multiple beneficial effects in the right doses at the right time, providing you don't expose yourself enough to burn your skin. In an ideal world, we should all expose at least our arms and legs (and, at times, our torso) to the sun for 10-20 minutes a day sometime between 11 am and 1 pm without sunscreen. If you have fair skin, make it 10 minutes, and if darker skinned, you may need to be exposed regularly for up to half an hour. While sunlight is essential for our skin to be able to manufacture its own vitamin D, regular exposure is also linked to improved mood, improved sleep, improved brain function, and preventing high blood pressure.[537] If you are lucky enough to be able to give yourself a short daily dose of sunlight, the take-home message is don't use sunscreen unless you want to stay out exposed to the sun for longer than 20-30 minutes.

About sunscreens
Sunscreens with 'non-nanoparticle' zinc oxide, titanium oxide, or avobenzone do a reasonable job at blocking both UV-A and UV-B. Other effective agents include ocryl-dimethy-PABA, octyl methoxy-cinnamate, 4 methyl-benzylidene camphor (4-MBC), octocrylene, benzophenone-3, homosalate, octisalate, octinoxate, and oxybenzone, but these are proving to be very harmful to the environment. Octinoxate and oxybenzone have been found to be particularly harmful to marine life, and these, along with several other suspect chemicals, are only now being banned to halt the environmental damage. Also, recent studies show that when sunscreen is applied to the skin, the chemicals in the sunscreen are absorbed and are found circulating in the bloodstream immediately after application.[538] We don't yet know of the short- and long-term health implications of this.

Low thyroid function and autoimmunity

Thyroid problems are more common in women than men, particularly at and after midlife.[36] I explained the nature of some of the thyroid issues seen in many midlife women on **pages 33 & 95**. Testing for thyroid problems is easy, although sometimes interpreting the test results is not straightforward, especially when your test looks normal, yet your symptoms match what would be expected if your thyroid was under functioning.

Clues that your thyroid function is not functioning optimally:

- tiredness and easy fatigue, especially in the afternoons
- dry, thinning hair and dry scalp
- thinning of the outer part of your eyebrows
- palpitations at rest (also in overactive thyroid)
- dry skin all over, but especially lower legs
- constipation
- a sudden increase in blood cholesterol.

In most women, the body tightly regulates the balance between the inactive form of thyroid hormone, called T4 and the *active* form of thyroid hormone, called T3. This balance keeps the body's metabolism functioning optimally. In 5-10% of women, the conversion from T4 to T3 is 'slower' than normal and this may result in them experiencing symptoms of low thyroid function as outlined in the text box above. These women can often benefit from specific T3 replacement medication (most thyroid medications are in the form of T4), despite having normal thyroid function on blood testing. The conversion from T4 to T3 can also be slowed down by a number of factors in any woman, and I have outlined these in the text box below.

Factors that reduce active T3 in the body:

- acute and chronic severe illness
- severe inflammation for any reason, including mold-exposure
- trauma and severe stress
- erratic estrogen levels (midlife)
- estrogen-related increase in T3-binding hormones
- deficiency in iron, iodine, zinc or selenium
- medications, e.g., amiodarone and lithium carbonate.

If your thyroid function test looks normal, have your healthcare provider check you for deficiencies in iron, iodine, selenium and zinc. Also check in with yourself as to whether you need to reduce whole-body inflammation or stress. If you continue to be concerned, ask your healthcare provider to check you for thyroid autoimmunity. This involves checking whether you have thyroid antibodies or a positive ANA (anti-nuclear antibody). If you turn out to have positive thyroid antibodies or a positive ANA, you should also check your vitamin D level, because low vitamin D is linked to autoimmunity. If you think that you may be one of those people that could benefit from a trial of thyroid therapy, seek out a healthcare provider versed in the nuances of thyroid hormone therapy.

Tips to reduce inflammation and autoimmunity:

- reduce your exposure to xenoestrogens (Estrogen Clearing Program)
- avoid high lectin foods including nightshades
- check your vitamin D and selenium levels
- if stressed, focus on relaxation techniques (Basic Program)
- if you have persistent inflammatory symptoms, check your house or office for water-damage and mold.

The Solutions

Targeted Solutions (3):

- Hot flushes and night sweats
- Menopausal hormone therapy (MHT)
- Vaginal dryness and atrophy
- Vaginal infections
- Urinary tract infections
- Painful bladder syndrome

Hot flushes and night sweats

Hot flushes and night sweats are the hallmark of Zone 4, but as I explained in **Section Two**, sometimes they can start as early as Zone 1. If you are going to get severe hot flushes, you will probably start to feel them by Zone 3. They tend to be at their worst during the six or so months before reaching Zone 4 and for 12-24 months after. If you do start experiencing flushing in Zone 1, you might notice that it is worse during the week before your menstrual period or at midcycle.[178] This indicates that your flushing may be due to large swings in your hormone levels rather than a loss of hormones. Importantly, if you are in Zone 1 or Zone 2 and your flushing and sweats are only at night and are the same throughout your cycle, you should consult your healthcare provider to get checked for other possible causes of the night sweats.

Useful tips that can help reduce flushing:

- keep cool (physically and mentally), dress in layers
- use cool bedding and sheets
- notice the things that trigger your flushing
- investigate a 'cooling pad' to sleep on
- avoid outdoor intense exercise, especially on hot days
- lose weight if you know you need to
- focus on reducing your stress
- reduce or stop alcohol.

Stopping alcohol may not help reduce flushing in some women. If you use alcohol to relieve excess stress, stopping alcohol could worsen your flushes. If this is you, alcohol is likely to be taking the edge off your flushing and/or sweats by relieving the symptoms of stress. This isn't an ideal long-term solution, so to reduce your alcohol intake without affecting your flushes, follow the Basic Program to reduce excess inflammation and stress.

Management strategies for hot flushes according to your Zone

Zone 1

Ask your healthcare provider about 150-200 mg oral progesterone taken before bed every night except on menstrual cycle days 1-7 (stop taking it during your menstrual period). Progesterone cream may add some benefit to the oral progesterone if you have severe PMS symptoms, especially anxiety. In this case, discuss a trial of 2.5-5% progesterone cream with your healthcare provider applied every night before bed except on menstrual cycle days 1-7.

Figure 12: Flow chart for hot flush management in Zone 1

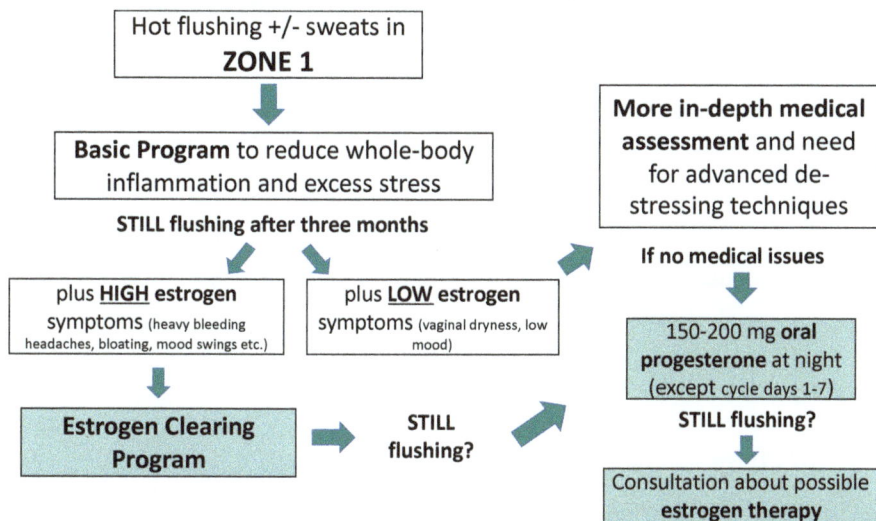

Zone 2 and Zone 3

The approach to hot flushing in Zone 2 and Zone 3 will depend on whether you have any other symptoms, and whether these symptoms indicate you have high or low estrogen. In Zone 3, it is common to experience both high and low estrogen symptoms. In both Zone 2 and Zone 3 women, I suggest starting off with the Basic Program. If you have symptoms of low estrogen (hot flushes or sleep disturbance), I would start transdermal estrogen therapy along with the Basic Program. If you don't have symptoms of low estrogen, I would continue the Basic Program and consider adding 150-200 mg oral progesterone before bed if sleep disturbance is an issue.

If symptoms persist or you are concerned about the symptoms, I would suggest further stress-reduction techniques and consider cautiously increasing the dose of estrogen. No two women respond the same way or the same extent to the diet, lifestyle, medication, or hormonal interventions, so judicious trial and error is key.

I rarely prescribe synthetic progestins in place of progesterone in hormone therapy, as these can have significant side effects, may increase the risk of breast cancer, and may offset the possible beneficial effects of estrogen on the heart.[359] Moreover, synthetic progestins are not as beneficial for night sweats or disrupted sleep. Also, as previously mentioned on **page 170**, progesterone cream is ineffective in reducing severe hot flushes in Zone 3 and Zone 4 women. It may however be beneficial in reducing mild cyclical flushing in some Zone 1 and Zone 2 women. Progesterone cream shouldn't be used in Zone 3 or Zone 4 to counteract the effect of estrogen therapy on the endometrium.

Zone 4

When you have reached Zone 4 and have significant hot flushes and night sweats, you have entered into world of Menopausal Hormone Therapy (MHT). Menopausal hot flushes remain the main indication for starting treatment with menopausal hormone therapy,[539] although it is also beneficial for bones, and in my experience, it will often benefit other symptoms that are common in menopause including low mood, emotional lability, muscle/joint aches and pains, and quality of life.

Any time I prescribe estrogen therapy to a patient, I also teach them the principles of the Estrogen Clearing Program. This helps to optimize their ability to detoxify their own estrogen and the estrogen in MHT. It is possible that the estrogen in MHT, especially in high doses and for several decades, could be harmful. This is also why I prescribe the lowest effective dose of estrogen possible according to your symptoms. Before discussing MHT at length, I will cover some of the non-hormonal medications and other therapies.

If your flushing and sweating symptoms do not respond to any of the therapies outlined here, consult your healthcare provider. Don't forget to let them know if you have other poor health complaints, such as daytime fatigue, poor concentration, forgetfulness, poor vision, headaches, bloating, irregular bowel habits, poor motivation, or low mood. Some of the actions they might take include performing a thorough symptom history and arranging a series of blood tests for fasting glucose, insulin, homocysteine, cholesterol, triglycerides, lipoprotein(a), high-sensitive CRP, kidney and liver function testing including a 'GGT', iron studies, vitamin D, vitamin B12, thyroid function, thyroid antibodies and anti-nuclear antibody or 'ANA'. They may also include X-rays, ultrasounds or other radiology investigations.

Figure 13: Management according to Zone 2, Zone 3, and Zone 4

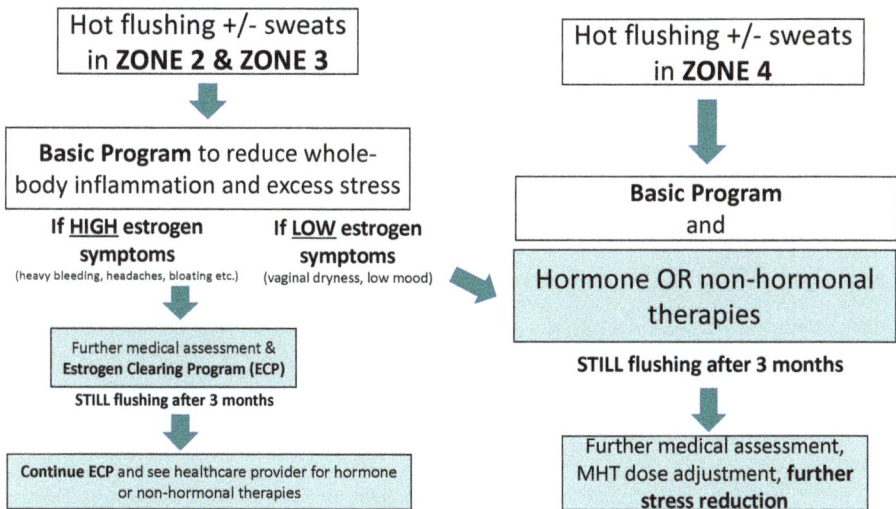

Should you treat your hot flushes or put up with them?

This is a good question. The research data on whether treating flushes with hormone therapy will benefit your overall health is extensive, contradictory, and therefore not conclusive. As a result, each 'expert' like myself will have their own opinion. My own understanding of the literature to date and my clinical experience leads me to advise all my Zone 4 patients with bothersome flushes and disrupted sleep to consider starting hormone or non-hormone therapy along with health-promoting programs including the Basic and Estrogen Clearing Programs. While we know that bothersome hot flushes are linked to having heart disease, we do not know yet for sure whether hot flush therapies will reverse some of the ill effects that severe hot flushes have on your future heart health.

Non-hormonal medical treatments

There are some medications including gabapentin, clonidine, and some anti-depressants that have been shown to be effective in reducing hot flushes, but they don't work as well as MHT. Another medication that was devised specifically for hot flushes called Fezolinetant works by blocking the KNDy cells in the hypothalamus in the brain. I explained what KNDy cells are on **page 82**. These non-hormonal medications are important options for women who have had breast cancer, have had other hormone-sensitive cancers or cannot tolerate hormone therapies. As with hormone therapies, I always prescribe them in combination with the principles of the Basic Program.

Non-hormonal treatments are less effective than hormone therapies at reducing hot flushes, so be aware that when taking these medications, you are aiming to have your flushing be a little less often, less severe, and less intrusive to daily activities and sleep. A further reduction in the severity of symptoms may be achieved through incorporating relaxation techniques, meditation, and some of the non-pharmaceutical therapies.

There is one other medication used in menopausal hot flushes called Tibolone. This medication is a selective tissue estrogenic regulator (STEAR) and although it isn't exactly an estrogen it can act like estrogen in the brain, bone and vagina. Thus, Tibolone is effective in reducing hot flushes and night sweats,[540] and it also helps maintain bone [541] and reduce vaginal dryness.[542]

Unlike other non-hormone medications, it cannot be used in women who have had breast cancer, because it has been linked to recurrence of the cancer and its safety as far as causing breast cancer remains uncertain.[543]

Non-pharmaceutical therapies

If you cannot or choose not to take hormone therapies or non-hormone medications, there are some plant-based therapies that might help. The most well-studied are on black cohosh[544] and red clover,[545] both plant-estrogens, also called phytoestrogens. Other options are less well studied and, while no clear improvement has been seen in research studies, in my experience, they can help women who are flushing feel better:

Non-pharmaceutical therapies:

Black cohosh	40-80 mg of root extract
Red clover	80-160 mg daily
St John's wort	300-600 mg 3 daily
Maca powder	1-2 tsp daily
Magnolia bark (honokil)[453]	50-200 mg 1-2 daily
Ashwagandha	500-1000 mg 2-3 daily
Passionflower extract	250-350 mg 1-2 daily

Menopausal or Zone 4 hormone therapy (MHT)

Is MHT the same as HRT and what does it involve?

Menopausal hormone therapy (MHT) refers to the hormone therapy prescribed in menopause, Zone 4. In the past, MHT was always referred to as hormone *replacement* therapy or HRT, however the 'R' for *replacement* has been dropped because the aim of MHT is to relieve symptoms rather than 'replace' what used to be there. It may take some years however for HRT to be replaced by MHT across the board.

MHT usually consists of estrogen alone (if you don't have a uterus), or in combination with a progestogen if you still have a uterus. A progestogen is the collective name for human equivalent progesterone therapies and synthetic forms of progestogens, called progestins. Progestogens are added to estrogen in MHT to protect your endometrium from building up too much in response to the estrogen. I prefer prescribing progesterone since it has fewer side effects than the synthetic progestins and in many women vastly improves sleep. Sometimes progesterone alone is prescribed for menopausal hot flushes, but it seems to be less effective than estrogen and requires high doses of around 300-400 mg daily.[546] As mentioned earlier, progesterone cream is not at all effective in reducing hot flushes or night sweats.

What to consider if you want to start MHT

Always consult your healthcare provider before taking hormone therapy so you can be fully assessed for contraindications, including breast and other cancers and blood clotting disorders. If you have been in Zone 4 more than 10 years and have never had estrogen therapy, you should see your healthcare provider before starting it. There are health risks associated with starting estrogen therapy more than 10 years after menopause, so you should consult your healthcare provider about getting a thorough health checkup and to discuss the possible risks. If you already have established heart disease or have significant risk factors for heart disease such as high blood pressure, obesity, pre-diabetes or diabetes, or high blood triglycerides, your healthcare provider may advise against it.

Assessing the long-term risks
In terms of all potential adverse effects, the risks of taking estrogen via a cream or a gel have not yet been fully defined, but they are likely to be lower than any form of oral estrogen. Regarding breast cancer risk, we know that including a synthetic progestin with estrogen is linked to an increased risk of breast cancer[547, 548] and cardiovascular disease.[549] This MHT combination is also

linked to an increased risk of cardiovascular disease.[550, 551] Oral estrogen alone looks to be linked to a lower risk of breast cancer in the long term and trans-dermal estrogen with or without oral progesterone so far looks to be neutral in terms of this risk.[552-554]

The research to date on taking long term estrogen alone, or estrogen and progesterone indicates that it is safe in terms of not significantly increasing your risk of getting other cancers[555] or heart disease[466]. The consensus is that estrogen-containing hormone therapy can be continued safely for at least 10 years, but emerging data will help your healthcare provider weigh up the risks of continuing it for longer. Meanwhile I believe it is very worthwhile combining any MHT with the Estrogen Clearing Program. It is also worthwhile working with your healthcare provider to determine the lowest dose of estrogen that is effective for you, while ensuring that dose will continue to benefit other parts of your body such as bone.

In Zone 4, after your ovaries stop producing high levels of estrogen and progesterone, your fat tissue starts to take over as the main source of estrogen. In general, the more fat tissue you have, the more estrogen (in the form of 'estrone') you produce. Estrone from fat tissue may help protect your bones but it doesn't seem to reduce your chance of getting menopausal symptoms. In fact, being obese is a risk factor for getting bothersome daytime and night-time hot flushes. Moreover, obesity is linked to a higher risk of getting breast cancer. I strongly suggest the Basic and Estrogen Clearing Programs if you have a body mass index of >30, particularly if you are taking MHT.

Should I include testosterone in my MHT?

Testosterone is occasionally added to MHT in the form of a cream or troche. The indications for testosterone with MHT include low blood levels that are accompanied by symptoms of low testosterone despite usual MHT. The symptoms of low testosterone are non-specific but include low libido, fatigue, muscle wasting, muscle weakness and inability to build muscle. Testosterone levels don't need to be routinely measured unless you have persistent bothersome symptoms that could indicate you have low testosterone. If levels were low, I would only recommend adding testosterone to your MHT if you had symptoms. There are also instances where women with low testosterone symptoms have blood levels that are considered to be within normal range, but they still feel a lot better taking testosterone.

When did MHT become available to women?

Hormone therapy began to change women's lives with the invention of the first birth control pills in the 1930s and 40s. By the 1960s, hormone therapy was being given to menopausal women for hot flushing. At the time, birth control hormones were synthesized in specialized laboratories from a plant cholesterol compound called diosgenin, a component of yam,[556] while the hormones used in MHT were 'harvested' from the urine of pregnant mares (called 'conjugated equine estrogens'). Why were menopausal hormones harvested from horses? The answer lies partly in the fact that relief of symptoms in menopausal women required higher doses than those used in the birth control pill. Another part of the answer at that time, had a lot to do with the substantial laboratory costs of manufacturing estrogen from diosgenin. Since the 1990s however, this cost has dramatically fallen. In addition, for a pharmaceutical product to be marketable, it had to be profitable and in order for it to be profitable, it has to be patentable. In order for it to be patentable, the product couldn't be a naturally occurring human hormone.

Although estrogen from horses could be described as 'natural' in that it isn't manufactured in a laboratory, the fact that it isn't a naturally occurring human hormone, meant it could be patented and therefore marketed. And so began the long and sorry story of pregnant mare urine (PMU) farms that produce horse estrogens for MHT. Nowadays, all human-equivalent female hormones including estrogen, progesterone and testosterone can be easily and efficiently produced in pharmaceutical laboratories from diosgenin. Despite these human-equivalent hormones being laboratory-synthesized, they are also often referred to as being 'natural' because they are *equivalent* to human estrogens and hormones. Note that while horse-urine derived 'conjugated estrogens' are also sometimes referred to as 'natural', they are obviously not 'human-equivalent'. Thus, the description of what is a 'natural' hormone has been a source of ongoing confusion. Pharmaceutical companies have been able to produce 'human-equivalent' estrogen and progesterone for decades, but because it wasn't profitable to sell them as commercial products until recently, they instead sold the hormones directly to *compounding* pharmacies. The compounding pharmacies in turn used these human-equivalent hormones to create custom-made hormone products, known as 'bio-identical hormones'.

We shouldn't forget about the horses

For the reasons I explained above, for several decades, horse estrogens were the only marketable FDA-approved estrogen available for MHT. As a result, pregnant mare urine (PMU) farms sprang up all over Canada, North America, South America, and even China. Unfortunately for horses, conjugated equine estrogens were chosen to be the MHT for women taking part in the $260 million Women's Health Initiative (WHI) study. I cannot help thinking that this decision represented a sizeable human failing and a huge step back for animal welfare. I say this because at the time, a laboratory-synthesized human-equivalent form of estrogen called estrogen valerate had already arrived on the market. This estrogen didn't require the killing and maiming of many thousands of perpetually pregnant mares and their foals. Estrogen valerate is a synthetic estrogen that after ingestion, is converted to human-equivalent estrogen.

Despite the economic viability and availability of laboratory-produced estrogens for MHT these days, conjugated equine estrogen from mares continues to be marketed world-wide in the form of estrogen creams, stand-alone estrogen capsules and in combination medications for bone health.[557] Nowadays, the estrogen from mares is simply referred to as conjugated estrogens instead of conjugated *equine* estrogens. Thus, these products no longer convey their origins, and women are not informed in any way that their MHT product comes from mare urine. I believe that if women knew that their MHT was derived from the urine of perpetually pregnant mares, most would say 'no thanks!' Hence the disappearance of 'equine' from the product labels.

There is no doubt that women have benefitted worldwide from the landmark WHI study which used equine estrogens. The study was stopped prematurely in 2002 due to concerns about the excess risks of breast cancer, stroke, and heart disease that were identified. It turns out, however, that equine estrogens alone (without a progestin) have an overall health benefit and that the health risks were only significant when combined with the progestin, medroxyprogesterone.[558] The cessation of the WHI unfortunately meant that many menopausal women who suffered severe menopausal symptoms were unable to access MHT from their healthcare providers. Many, however, sought out *bio-identical* MHT products produced by compounding pharmacies. This is when bio-identical MHT gained widespread popularity.

According to a small survey of women using bio-identical MHT, women said they chose bio-identical MHT for several reasons including not wanting to take mare urine products, their concerns about the problems seen in the WHI study, and their 'overarching distrust of a medical system which they perceived as dismissive of their concerns and overly reliant on pharmaceuticals'.[559]

It could have been a win for women and a win for horses if the dramatic fall in MHT use (after the WHI study had to be stopped) was followed by the replacement of horse urine estrogens with those produced in laboratories from diosgenin plants. There is now a large array of hormone therapy products that contain human-equivalent plant-derived estrogens, so there is no longer any practical or medical need for mare-derived estrogens. We can only hope that the removal of 'equine' on product labelling doesn't mean the horses are forgotten for good and will never be set free.

Bio-identical and body-identical MHT

The difference between the two has little to do with their names 'bio-' and 'body-' identical. They both contain human-equivalent estrogen and proges-terone hormones that come from the same place, a pharmaceutical laboratory.

While 'bio-identical' MHT *products* are made by compounding pharmacists, 'body-identical' MHT products are marketed and sold by pharmaceutical companies. So, they contain the same hormones derived from the same plant by the same pharmaceutical companies. The primary difference is 'body-identical' MHT products have been approved by regulatory bodies and packaged according to strict guidelines.

Bio-identical compounded MHT

One of the earliest bio-identical MHT products in use was called Tri-Est, a combination of three human-equivalent estrogens referred to as estrone (E1), estradiol (E2) and estriol (E3). The three estrogens were thought to create a more body-friendly estrogen therapy than giving estradiol, or E2, alone. The problem is that we can't be sure that it is really 'body-friendly' because these three estrogens are interchangeable within our bodies anyway (our bodies can convert one to another). In fact, few practitioners who prescribe bio-identical hormones today still use this Tri-Est combination, and most either use Bi-Est (various combinations of E2 and E3 without E1) or just E2 (estradiol) alone. Many advocates for bio-identical MHT products still believe that giving a combination of E2 and E3 is more 'physiological' and therefore better for the female body. Some also believe that the less potent E3 can offset the 'strength' of the more potent E2, but it makes more sense to me to simply reduce the dose of the E2. My advice is to start with an E2-only transdermal patch and if this is not suitable or is not available, compounded E2-alone cream or E2-alone gel.

Many practitioners who prescribe bio-identical MHT have been taught to monitor their patients' therapy using repeated salivary or urine hormone measurements. If this sounds like your practitioner, consider telling them that you don't need multiple expensive tests and that your symptoms are the best guide in working through the process of optimizing your hormone therapy. I occasionally check blood levels during MHT therapy, but I don't use repeated blood, urine or salivary hormone testing to monitor therapy. Finally, be aware that many practitioners who prescribe bio-identical E2/E3 or E2 creams also use progesterone creams to protect the endometrium. If this is the case, let them know that you need to take at least 100 mg of *oral* progesterone to guarantee safety in this regard. Vaginal progesterone is an alternative way to protect from endometrial build up, but this preparation is not commonly used in MHT.

If you are using bio-identical hormones or thinking about it, you need to know about compounding pharmacists, because they are the ones putting your product together. Compounding pharmacists were the original pharmacists. In fact, the art of pharmaceutical compounding came into being before modern medicine, and the pediatric, dermatology, and endocrinology professions have for many years, and still do depend on compounders to individualize doses for their patients. In Canada and Europe, many medical doctors work alongside compounding pharmacists, enabling them to individualize doses and formulations. In some countries like the US and Australia, however, most doctors have little knowledge of what compounding pharmacists offer, and most pharmacists don't learn anything about compounding. Learning to be a compounder is now only an option (not a core subject) in pharmacy training.

Despite the lack of awareness surrounding compounding pharmacists, they still play an important role in medicine and drug therapy because compounders can provide medications in doses and formulations that are not available in marketed pharmaceutical products. They also play a role if a previously used pharmaceutical product gets taken off the market but the drug/hormone within that product is still manufactured. This allows the pharmaceutical companies to produce the drug, sell it for profit, but not bear the exorbitant costs of manufacturing a strictly regulated product. In other words, the pharmaceutical companies can still 'do business' by providing the drug/hormone to compounders who then make the drug available to patients via their compounded capsules, liquids, or creams, etc.

One of the most important aspects of compounded products that I recently discovered is that they often create products that are free from added preservatives, colors, and other filler chemicals. Some of my most sensitive patients who cannot tolerate these additives are forever grateful for their compounded medications.

In terms of regulation, each country has unique pharmacy guidelines whereby pharmacists and their compounding laboratories can be certified in the process of creating reliable MHT and other products. Sometimes, these certification processes are not mandatory, so if you are using a compounded medication for any purpose, check that your compounding pharmacy has gone through and passed this process. The usual margin of error in dosing in a pharmaceutical product is said to be 1-2%, compared to 5-10% for a compounded product. This margin of error in compounded products is more important for some medications than others. For example, because estrogen circulates in the blood at much lower levels (measured in pg/mL) than progesterone (measured in ng/mL), the margin of error in compounded estrogen products is more important to consider than in compounded progesterone products. The margin of error will also likely increase when the compounded product is administered as a cream or an ointment. Estrogen's low margin of error is the reason why I am less likely to prescribe a compounded estrogen than a compounded progesterone. In addition, there are many more choices for pharmaceutical estrogen MHT products (patches, gels and tablets) than pharmaceutical progesterone MHT products (only 100 or 200 mg progesterone tablets).

Because compounded MHT products cannot be patented or standardized, they are hardly ever used in clinical research studies. Thus, I reserve compounded estrogen for women who cannot tolerate a pharmaceutical version, or for whom it is ineffective. For example, some women, who are allergic to the estrogen patches and gels may do better with a compounded body cream or a vaginal cream. While I don't recommend the use of troches because of the inconsistency in absorption, there are some women who have tried everything else without success.

Transdermal vs. oral estrogens in MHT

For many decades, the only estrogen-containing MHT medications were tablets. When compared to transdermal estrogen MHT, oral estrogen

MHT carries a higher risk of blood clotting, stroke and heart disease.[560, 561] Compounding pharmacists have been creating transdermal estrogen MHT products since the 1960-1970s (creams and gels) but it wasn't until the mid-eighties, when the pharmaceutical industry followed suit by marketing the first transdermal estrogen patches. This technology allowed pharmaceutical companies to successfully market human-equivalent estrogens because they could patent their delivery system rather than the estrogen itself.

Since the mid-90s, the variety of transdermal MHT products containing human-equivalent estrogen has expanded and now these products make up the bulk of the estrogen containing MHT market share. Studies have shown that transdermal estrogen patches deliver precise and constant levels of estrogen[562] and patches have become the preferred option over all other delivery systems such as gels, creams and tablets.[554, 562] Examples include EstraDerm®, Estradot®, Estelle®, and Climara®.

There are no data on estrogen delivered via a compounded cream and data for estrogen gels are just emerging now.[563, 564] In general, estrogen containing gels and creams don't deliver as precise of a level of estrogen and gels in particular deliver the estrogen to the bloodstream rapidly rather than in a slow-release fashion. This fast release may adversely affect their safety profile because of the large delivery of hormone to the blood and then the liver.

Body-identical progesterone

As I have outlined before, if you still have a uterus and are on estrogen-containing MHT, you need progesterone or a synthetic progestin to counteract the estrogen-induced build-up within the endometrium. If estrogen is taken on its own, it can increase the future risk of endometrial cancer, a risk that is proportionate to the dose and length of estrogen therapy. The only option that women had for many years were synthetic progestins, and it wasn't until recently that an oral form of human-equivalent progesterone became widely available. Synthetic progestins include those used in birth control pills, like desogestrel, norethindrone, norgestel, and drogesterone, and those used in

MHT, like levonorgestrel, norethisterone, and medroxyprogesterone.

The synthetic progestin components of MHT seem to significantly contribute to the adverse side effects of MHT, including abnormal blood clotting, cardiovascular disease, stroke, increased breast cancer risk, and mood problems. They can also cause troublesome symptoms including fluid retention, headache, loss of libido, and weight gain. In fact, synthetic progestins have no therapeutic effects outside of endometrial protection. On the other hand, human-equivalent progesterone has additional therapeutic effects including its ability to improve disturbed sleep.[411] It also plays a role in the maintenance of healthy bone and may be linked to a lower risk of breast cancer, heart disease, and mood disorders when compared to the synthetic progestins.[565]

When delivered orally in a micronized capsule, progesterone benefits sleep through its main breakdown product, called allopregnanolone. This compound has multiple positive effects on the brain, including a calming effect via GABA receptors, and as stated in one scientific review:

Progesterone plays a myriad of roles in neurophysiological homeostasis and adaptation to stress while exerting anxiolytic, antidepressant, antinociceptive, anticonvulsant, anti-inflammatory, sleep promoting, memory stabilizing, neuroprotective, pro-myelinating, and neurogenic effects.[566]

In my practice, I prescribe both the pharmaceutical and compounded versions of progesterone capsules. Compounded versions are useful for women who either cannot tolerate the pharmaceutical product (contains titanium dioxide, DNC red color #10, and FDNC yellow color #6), or need a dose different to those supplied by the pharmaceutical product. Progesterone has been available in 100 and 200 mg capsules in the USA and Europe for more than 15 years and has also been approved in Australia and the UK. Transdermal progesterone patches are not yet available and, given the high doses required in MHT, they are unlikely to be in future. Progesterone cream does not play a role in MHT but as I have discussed, it can be used in the short-term for some symptoms experienced by women in Zone 1, Zone 2, and Zone 3.

Talk to your health provider about MHT if you:

- have hot flushing or night sweats in Zone 3 or Zone 4
- have reached Zone 4 before or around age 45
- have reached Zone 4 and have a family history of osteoporosis, or have risk factors for osteoporosis
- are interested in taking MHT for any reason.

Caution is needed when considering MHT if:

- you have been in Zone 4 for >10 years
- you or a family member has had breast cancer or other hormone-dependent cancer
- you have had a blood clot in the leg, arm, or lung
- you cannot take HT for medical reasons and need to explore non-hormonal treatments.

Vaginal dryness and vaginal atrophy

Vaginal dryness can be an extremely troubling symptom, especially in sexually active midlife and menopausal women. If left untreated, it can lead to a painful condition known as vaginal atrophy, or *atrophic vulvo-vaginitis. Atrophy* refers to the loss of, or shrinkage of the mucous membranes, muscles, and connective tissue inside and outside the vagina. There is also shrinkage of surrounding organs (bladder, urethra, etc.) and their support structures. This, in turn, can lead to vaginal and pelvic pain, inability to have intercourse and an increased likelihood of vaginal prolapse and urinary infections.

The most effective treatment for vaginal dryness and atrophy is hormone therapy applied as a cream, a gel, or a pessary. The hormones that are most commonly used in gels and creams are estriol, estradiol, and DHEA. Most of the pharmaceutical pessary products contain estriol, but estradiol, estriol and DHEA have been shown to reverse the symptoms of vaginal dryness and atrophy. Recently both DHEA and estriol vaginal creams have been shown to improve sexual function.[567, 568] Estriol has also been found to improve the health of the vaginal microbiome,[569] and when combined with the probiotic lactobacillus, has been effective in managing severe symptoms.[570] The success of this combination makes sense as the lactobacillus bacteria produce glycogen which promotes the health of the inner vaginal walls and reduces the populations of harmful bacteria.[571]

Use of topical vaginal estrogen creams can cause a slight rise in blood levels of estrogen, but it depends on the dose in the preparation and frequency of use. In general, only about 20% of any estriol applied intravaginally via a cream, gel, or pessary reaches the circulation.[572] If you have a history of breast cancer or other hormone-dependent cancer, check with your cancer specialist before using any of these preparations. There is growing evidence that vaginal estrogen is not linked to breast cancer recurrence in survivors,[573-575] however most cancer specialists still only allow DHEA cream or gel. DHEA cream or gel doesn't cause any estrogen-like actions in the body and doesn't increase DHEA (or other hormone) levels in the blood.[568] For advanced cases of vaginal atrophy, creams and gels are probably more effective than pessaries, but it is a personal choice. I find vaginal cream with a combination of E3 (estriol) and DHEA is very effective even if vaginal atrophy is severe. The cream is used daily for 2-3 weeks, then it can be reduced to three times a week, which is the usual 'maintenance dose'.

Vaginal lubricants

Lubricants are used as alternatives to topical hormones for vaginal dryness and/or vaginal atrophy in menopause but can be used for general intercourse 'accessories' at any age. Lubricants are usually water-based or silicon-based creams or gels that make the vaginal entrance and surrounding areas slippery. If you are in Zone 4 and have vaginal dryness however, lubricants have the potential to *increase* discomfort during intercourse. If you make intercourse with a dry vagina more feasible by making it more 'slippery', you may be causing more abrasions and/or micro-tears inside and around the vagina. It follows that this would be more likely if the vaginal mucosa and surrounding structures are atrophied. So, if you have a dry atrophied vagina, the most effective treatments would be those that improve the health and function of the vaginal mucous membranes and surrounding muscle/tissue structures.

Recurrent vaginal infections, vaginosis, vaginal thrush

If you get repeated vaginal infections (vaginosis) or vaginal thrush, it is an indication that the vaginal mucous membranes lining your vagina may not be as healthy as they could be and may not be supporting a healthy population of lactobacillus bacteria. So, while it is important to treat infections, it is equally important to add treatments that help restore a healthy resident bacteria population. Talk to your healthcare provider about the treatment options.

> **Treatment options for vaginal infections:**
> - single course of metronidazole or tinidazole
> - 0.2-1% hydrogen peroxide[576] douches for 3 days, then weekly until fully cleared
> - 300-600 mg boric acid[577] compounded vaginal cream daily for 1-2 weeks, then weekly until fully cleared.

Metronidazole and tinidazole are antibiotics that are active against most of the organisms that cause vaginosis. These antibiotics are generally well tolerated but can cause nausea and recurrent vaginal thrush (candida overgrowth and/or infection).[578] As a result, some women prefer topical antimicrobial douches and addressing ways to improve the vaginal microbiome.[579-581]

Hydrogen peroxide douches

Hydrogen peroxide or H_2O_2 douches are best performed while showering. Before showering, prepare 5-10 mL of 0.5-1% hydrogen peroxide solution and place it where you can access it while showering. If you use anything greater than a 1% solution, it is likely to sting. Using a 2-5 mL syringe, draw up some of your pre-prepared H_2O_2 solution, place the tip of the syringe 2-3 cm inside the opening of the vagina and gently plunge the syringe to slowly deliver the solution into the vagina. You can repeat this 1-2 times. Don't plunge the solution in quickly or suddenly. If you experience stinging sensations using the H_2O_2 solution you have prepared, try a more dilute solution, for example 0.2%. Once you have used this more dilute solution for a day or two, you may be able to increase it again to the target concentration of between 0.5 and 1%. Pharmacies usually have 3% H_2O_2 solutions available for purchase. You can re-use the syringes by thoroughly washing the syringe with warm soapy water inside and out after use.

Boric acid pessaries

This is a little-known treatment for recurrent vaginal infections but it has been shown to be around 80% effective in both one-time or recurrent vaginal bacterial and thrush infections.[577] Boric acid vaginal pessaries contain 300-600 mg boric acid and are available through compounding chemists. Note that the dose of boric acid in the pessary is about 100-fold higher than doses that are recommended for oral supplementation of boron (I discuss this in the 'Bones' section on **page 219**). Boron is well absorbed when taken orally, but if put on the skin or inside the vagina, it is only minimally absorbed. Nevertheless, it is worth knowing that a toxic dose of Boron is considered to be 20-80 g orally, more than 100 times the amount in a vaginal dose of 300-600 mg. Thus, it is safer than most household products as far as accidental ingestion. As with the H_2O_2 solutions, hormone creams, and toxic household products, keep the boric acid pessaries in a safe place away from prying young hands.

Treatment options to prevent recurrence of bacterial vaginosis

If you have recurrent vaginal bacterial infections, there is likely an underlying cause. It usually has something to do with the lack of health within your resident vaginal bacteria and their inability to fight off invasive, infection-promoting bacteria.[582] I would recommend a combination of a non-antibiotic topical treatment (e.g., H_2O_2 douche) in addition to an oral probiotic containing lactobacillus rhamnosus and/or lactobacillus reuteri 1-2 times a day until complete resolution.[580] Sometimes a lactobacillus probiotic capsule directly into the vagina is also needed. Thereafter, improving gut health through the Basic Program, oral probiotics and prebiotic fibers will in most cases prevent ongoing recurrence. I also advise stopping any habitual practices like vaginal douching or use of 'vaginal deodorants' as these greatly disrupt the healthy vaginal flora.

Recurrent urinary tract infections (recurrent cystitis or UTI)

If you have had recurrent cystitis, you have likely had to take repeated courses of antibiotics. As you may know, repeated courses of antibiotics can disrupt the healthy bacteria in your bowel. This disruption unfortunately has the potential to increase the risk of having further episodes of cystitis. Thus, for anyone with recurrent UTI's, in addition to necessary courses of antibiotics, I recommend a daily lactobacillus probiotic and 20-30 g of mixed supplementary fibers.[583] If after a month or so, you are still getting recurrent UTIs, talk to your health-care provider about adding a rectal dose of the lactobacillus probiotic. One of the best fiber supplements for boosting the numbers and health of gut/vaginal lactobacillus is a sticky liquid called lactulose. Lactulose is a sweet-tasting liquid that is often used in constipation. It cannot be absorbed by your intestines (zero calories for your body), and it passes through to the large bowel where it feeds all sorts of healthy bacteria including lactobacillus and bifidobacteria. If you get loose bowels from taking 5 mL twice a day, reduce the dose until the bowels settle. You can then try increasing it again slowly over a month or so.

Bladder pain syndrome (interstitial cystitis)

Bladder pain syndrome (BPS) is a 'diagnosis of exclusion' meaning your doctor will only be able to make the diagnosis if they have excluded infection or other physical causes of the pain. Many women with this diagnosis have often had repeated courses of antibiotics for presumed UTIs. The diagnosis requires a cystoscopy by a urology specialist to exclude other bladder problems, and during this procedure a biopsy of the bladder wall is taken. If there is bladder pain syndrome, the biopsies will reveal that the walls of the bladder are 'inflamed'. Some astute urologists may request special mast-cell-staining tests on the bladder biopsies to confirm or deny the presence of excess mast cells in the wall of the bladder. This is useful because the pain can be lessened with the use of anti-mast-cell medication.

BPS is poorly responsive to usual analgesic medications such as paracetamol and narcotics like morphine, or antidepressants like amitriptyline. When used in combination with anti-mast cell medication like H1-blockers and antihistamines, however, the pain can be better managed. Pelvic floor 'Kegel' exercises can also be helpful for some women who also have pelvic floor problems, but they are usually only effective for bladder pain when used in combination with carefully selected medications. The women who I have treated with BPS have also responded well to a low-oxalate diet. These women have usually had multiple courses of antibiotics and as a result, have lost a lot of their beneficial gut flora. This is often accompanied by a loss of the ability to break down dietary oxalates. One of the gut bacteria that is involved in the breakdown of oxalates in the diet is aptly named 'oxalobacter'. High oxalate levels are also linked to painful vagina syndrome, also called 'vulvodynia'. Vulvodynia can be abolished with the combination of a low oxalate diet and a broad-spectrum prebiotic fiber supplement. A low oxalate diet involves reducing high oxalate-containing foods like spinach (raw or cooked), rhubarb, soy, nuts, and tofu, and eating less food that contains moderate amounts; such foods include beans, black eyed peas, white or sweet potato with skins, beets, soy, miso soup, bamboo shoots, okra, bran, almonds, cashews, and dried fruits.

CLOSING THOUGHTS

Now that you have reached the end of this book, I hope that you have clarity regarding what to expect prior to, during and after the transition to menopause. It was always my intention to help you understand the key mind/body/hormone science that underpins successful management of midlife changes and symptoms. By conveying this knowledge, I want to help you feel more at ease and grounded in your body, so that you can better navigate your future health journey.

Whatever level of mastery you can achieve during your health journey, you will most likely require some input from a medical doctor or other healthcare provider. When seeking their advice and considering treatment options, it is important to clearly communicate your concerns and informed perspectives. Let them know you've educated yourself enough to engage in meaningful discussions. If you feel unheard, stay calm, reconnect with your needs, and determine whether to pursue further dialogue with them or seek another provider.

Honoring your intuitive wisdom extends beyond striving for optimal health. It is also about discovering your life purpose and fulfilling your potential in this world. This discovery process will likely improve your wellbeing, enrich your outlook and elevate your quality of life. Furthermore, your intuitive gifts will foster peace in place of war, nurturing in place of coercion and bullying, and creative humanity in place of soulless and inflexible dogma. In today's challenging times, these gifts are invaluable. Thank you for reading and God bless every one of you.

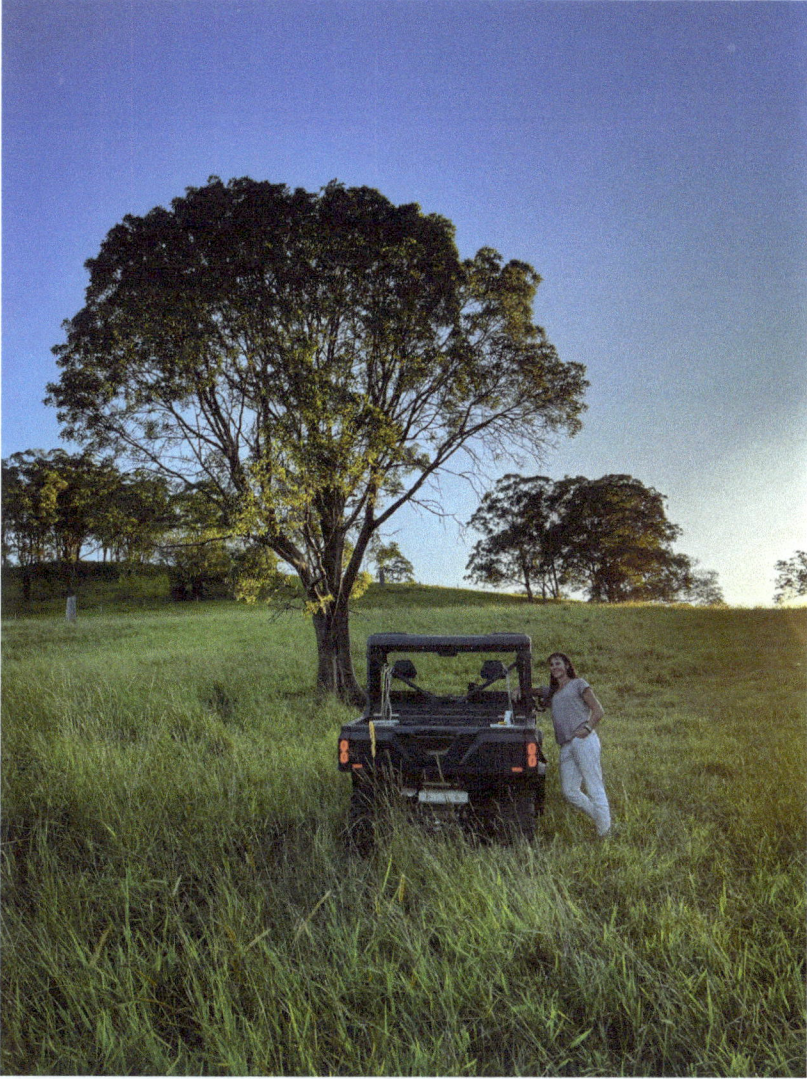

Thank you for reading and wishing you all the very best of health and happiness

ACKNOWLEDGEMENTS

Professor Ian S. Fraser: As my Ph.D. supervisor, Ian was simply a gift from God. Although no longer with us, what an incredible researcher and clinician he was. He allowed me to carry out my rather ambitious but key women's health study at the University of Sydney – the scientific basis for this book. I am greatly saddened that he cannot review and discuss this book with me.

Australasian Menopause Society: I couldn't be more grateful to the AMS who provided most of the funding for my Ph.D. study. As a previous board member, I can state that this organisation is fully committed to the wellbeing of midlife women in Australasia. Thank you.

Professor Claude L. Hughes: It was the bubbly and extremely talented Claude at the Cedars Sinai Medical Centre who helped me devise the study plan for my Ph.D. – a plan that allowed us to reveal the secrets of midlife menstrual cycle irregularities within 'LOOP' cycles.

Professor Noel Bairey Merz: A wonderful friend and unique researcher, Noel provided an important research environment at the Cedars Sinai Medical Centre to consolidate my Ph.D. research plan once back in Sydney.

Emeritus Professor Henry Burger: Henry, a life-long family friend and celebrated pioneer researcher in reproductive endocrinology. His support for my

Ph.D. and the results was so very much appreciated. His recent passing rocked me. I will miss him greatly. What a wonderful man.

Frank Manconi: Frank provided the all-important information and skills to analyse the menstrual blood loss outcomes in my Ph.D. at the University of Sydney. Frank is a uniquely kind-hearted, gentle person. Thank you, Frank.

Alison O'Dwyer: The production of this book has taken years and many twists and turns. I don't know what I would have done without Alison. Her eagle-eye and incredible attention to detail is second to none. I am honored to have her as a close and trusted friend. She is a unique, beautiful person.

Angela Thomas: To my gutsy, smart, savvy assistant and friend, thank you!

Friends and family: Thank you for your support and keeping my feet solidly on the ground to get this book done.

To all of my patients: You are amazing, you teach me new things every day. Here's to all of you!

Finally, huge gratitude to all the women who participated in my University of Sydney Ph.D. study. My sincere apologies for taking so long to get this book finished and 'out there'. Please contact me for a free copy of this book.

Appendix I:

THE STRAW+10 STAGING SYSTEM

The Zones' correspondences with the STRAW+10 stages:
- Zone 1 = **late reproductive age** = Straw Stage -3b and -3a
- Zone 2 = **early perimenopause** = Straw Stage -2
- Zone 3 = **late perimenopause** = Straw stage -1 and +1a
- Zone 4 = **menopause** = Straw Stage +1b and beyond

NOTE: because determining your Zone requires a functioning menstrual cycle, you can't determine your Zone if you have had your uterus removed (hysterectomy), have had longstanding and ongoing highly irregular cycles, or have other medical reasons that you have interrupted menstrual cycles.

Dr Georgina Hale, MD, Ph.D.

Table A: 'Your Zone' is based on the STRAW+10 staging system

FIRST menstrual period →

FINAL menstrual period →

STAGE	-5	-4	-3b	-3a	-2	-1	+1a	+1b	+1c	+2
Terminology	Reproductive				Menopausal transition		Postmenopause			
	Early	Peak		Late	Early	Late		Early		Late
					Perimenopause				Menopause	
Duration			Variable		Variable	1-3 yrs	2 yrs (1+1 yrs)		3-6 yrs	Lifespan
PRINCIPLE CRITERIA – TYPICAL MENSTRUAL CYCLE CHANGES										
Typical menstrual cycle changes	Variable-regular	Regular	Regular	Regular (subtle changes in flow and length)	Variable length (>7 day difference in cycle length)	Skipped cycles (>60 days between bleeds)				
YOUR ZONE			ZONE 1		ZONE 2		ZONE 3		ZONE 4	
Supportive endocrine testing criteria										
FSH			Low	Variable	↑ Variability	↑ >25 IU/L*	Mild high	Mod high	Very high	
AMH			Low	Low	Low	Low	Low	Low	Very low	
Inhibin B (INHB)			–	Low	Low	Low	Low	Low	Very low	
Antral follicles			Low	Low	Low	Low	Very Low	Very Low	Very low	Absent
Symptoms						Hot flushes, night sweats most likely here			Uro-genital problems here (vaginal dryness/atrophy)	

Adapted from Harlow et al.[584]

REFERENCES

1. Hansen, K.R., et al., *A new model of reproductive aging: the decline in ovarian non-growing follicle number from birth to menopause.* Human Reproduction, 2008. **23**(3): p. 699-708.
2. Yoshihara, M., et al., *The Continued Absence of Functional Germline Stem Cells in Adult Ovaries.* Stem Cells, 2023. **41**(2): p. 105-110.
3. Marcozzi, S., et al., *Programmed cell death in the human ovary.* Minerva Ginecol, 2018. **70**(5): p. 549-560.
4. Baerwald, A.R., G.P. Adams, and R.A. Pierson, *Characterization of Ovarian Follicular Wave Dynamics in Women.* Biology of Reproduction, 2003. **69**(3): p. 1023-1031.
5. Stringer, J.M., et al., *Beyond apoptosis: evidence of other regulated cell death pathways in the ovary throughout development and life.* Hum Reprod Update, 2023. **29**(4): p. 434-456.
6. Zhou, J., X. Peng, and S. Mei, *Autophagy in Ovarian Follicular Development and Atresia.* Int J Biol Sci, 2019. **15**(4): p. 726-737.
7. Lliberos, C., et al., *The Inflammasome Contributes to Depletion of the Ovarian Reserve During Aging in Mice.* Front Cell Dev Biol, 2020. **8**: p. 628473.
8. Titus, S., et al., *Individual-oocyte transcriptomic analysis shows that genotoxic chemotherapy depletes human primordial follicle reserve in vivo by triggering proapoptotic pathways without growth activation.* Sci Rep, 2021. **11**(1): p. 407.
9. Xu, Y.Q., et al., *[Female genital toxicities of high-frequency electromagnetic field on rats].* Zhonghua Lao Dong Wei Sheng Zhi Ye Bing Za Zhi, 2009. **27**(9): p. 544-8.
10. van Zonneveld, P., et al., *Do cycle disturbances explain the age-related decline of female fertility? Cycle characteristics of women aged over 40 years compared with a reference population of young women.* Human Reproduction, 2003. **18**(3): p. 495-501.

11. Scheffer, G.J., et al., *The number of antral follicles in normal women with proven fertility is the best reflection of reproductive age.* Human Reproduction, 2003. **18**(4): p. 700-6.

12. Hale, G.E., et al., *Endocrine features of menstrual cycles in middle and late reproductive age and the menopausal transition classified according to the Staging of Reproductive Aging Workshop (STRAW) staging system.* Journal of Clinical Endocrinology & Metabolism, 2007. **92**(8): p. 3060-7.

13. Soules, M.R., et al., *Stages of Reproductive Aging Workshop (STRAW).* Journal of Womens Health & Gender-Based Medicine, 2001. **10**(9): p. 843-8.

14. Santoro, N., et al., *Impaired folliculogenesis and ovulation in older reproductive aged women.* Journal of Clinical Endocrinology & Metabolism, 2003. **88**(11): p. 5502-9.

15. Klein, N.A., et al., *Ovarian follicular development and the follicular fluid hormones and growth factors in normal women of advanced reproductive age.* Journal of Clinical Endocrinology & Metabolism, 1996. **81**(5): p. 1946-51.

16. Klein, N.A., et al., *Is the short follicular phase in older women secondary to advanced or accelerated dominant follicle development?* Journal of Clinical Endocrinology & Metabolism, 2002. **87**(12): p. 5746-50.

17. Baerwald, A., et al., *Age-related changes in luteal dynamics: preliminary associations with antral follicular dynamics and hormone production during the human menstrual cycle.* Menopause, 2018. **25**(4): p. 399-407.

18. Coslov, N., M.K. Richardson, and N.F. Woods, *Symptom experience during the late reproductive stage and the menopausal transition: observations from the Women Living Better survey.* Menopause, 2021. **28**(9): p. 1012-1025.

19. Fanchin, R., et al., *Serum anti-Mullerian hormone is more strongly related to ovarian follicular status than serum inhibin B, estradiol, FSH and LH on day 3.* Human Reproduction, 2003. **18**(2): p. 323-7.

20. Anderson, R.A., S.M. Nelson, and W.H.B. Wallace, *Measuring anti-Mullerian hormone for the assessment of ovarian reserve: when and for whom is it indicated?* Maturitas, 2012. **71**(1): p. 28-33.

21. Hale, G.E., et al., *Atypical estradiol secretion and ovulation patterns caused by luteal out-of-phase (LOOP) events underlying irregular ovulatory menstrual cycles in the menopausal transition.* Menopause, 2009. **16**(1): p. 50-9.

22. Prior, J.C., et al., *Ovulation Prevalence in Women with Spontaneous Normal-Length Menstrual Cycles - A Population-Based Cohort from HUNT3, Norway.* PLoS One, 2015. **10**(8): p. e0134473.

23. Prior, J.C., S. Shirin, and A. Goshtasebi, *Bone health and prevalent fractures in women with polycystic ovary syndrome: a meta-analysis and endocrine-context pathophysiology review.* Expert Rev Endocrinol Metab, 2023. **18**(4): p. 283-293.

24. Seifert-Klauss, V., et al., *Progesterone and bone: a closer link than previously realized.* Climacteric, 2012. **15 Suppl 1**: p. 26-31.

25. Toffoletto, S., et al., *Emotional and cognitive functional imaging of estrogen and progesterone effects in the female human brain: a systematic review.* Psychoneuroendocrinology, 2014. **50**: p. 28-52.
26. Vollenhoven, B. and S. Hunt, *Ovarian ageing and the impact on female fertility.* F1000Res, 2018. **7**.
27. Guimarães, R.M., et al., *Oocyte Morphology and Reproductive Outcomes - Case Report and Literature Review.* JBRA Assist Reprod, 2021. **25**(3): p. 500-507.
28. Asprey, L.A., D., *the Better Baby book.* 2013, USA: Wiley.
29. Skiba, M.A., et al., *Androgens During the Reproductive Years: What Is Normal for Women?* J Clin Endocrinol Metab, 2019. **104**(11): p. 5382-5392.
30. Lasley, B.L., et al., *The relationship of circulating dehydroepiandrosterone, testosterone, and estradiol to stages of the menopausal transition and ethnicity.* Journal of Clinical Endocrinology & Metabolism, 2002. **87**(8): p. 3760-7.
31. Couzinet, B., et al., *The postmenopausal ovary is not a major androgen-producing gland.* J Clin Endocrinol Metab, 2001. **86**(10): p. 5060-6.
32. Sam, S. and D.A. Ehrmann, *Metformin therapy for the reproductive and metabolic consequences of polycystic ovary syndrome.* Diabetologia, 2017. **60**(9): p. 1656-1661.
33. Hale, G.E., C.L. Hughes, and J.M. Cline, *Clinical review 139 - Endometrial cancer: Hormonal factors, the perimenopausal "window of risk," and isoflavones [Review].* Journal of Clinical Endocrinology & Metabolism, 2002. **87**(1): p. 3-15.
34. Newman, M., et al., *Evaluating urinary estrogen and progesterone metabolites using dried filter paper samples and gas chromatography with tandem mass spectrometry (GC-MS/MS).* BMC chemistry, 2019. **13**(1): p. 20-20.
35. Thurston, R.C., *Vasomotor symptoms and cardiovascular health: findings from the SWAN and the MsHeart/MsBrain studies.* Climacteric, 2024. **27**(1): p. 75-80.
36. Ragusa, F., et al., *Hashimotos' thyroiditis: Epidemiology, pathogenesis, clinic and therapy.* Best Pract Res Clin Endocrinol Metab, 2019. **33**(6): p. 101367.
37. Mazokopakis, E.E., et al., *Is vitamin D related to pathogenesis and treatment of Hashimoto's thyroiditis?* Hell J Nucl Med, 2015. **18**(3): p. 222-7.
38. Stamatelopoulos, K.S., et al., *Arterial stiffness but not intima-media thickness is increased in euthyroid patients with Hashimoto's thyroiditis: The effect of menopausal status.* Thyroid, 2009. **19**(8): p. 857-62.
39. Koehler, V.F., N. Filmann, and W.A. Mann, *Vitamin D Status and Thyroid Autoantibodies in Autoimmune Thyroiditis.* Horm Metab Res, 2019. **51**(12): p. 792-797.
40. Zhang, C.Y., et al., *Abnormal uterine bleeding patterns determined through menstrual tracking among participants in the Apple Women's Health Study.* Am J Obstet Gynecol, 2023. **228**(2): p. 213.e1-213.e22.
41. Verrilli, L. and S.L. Berga, *What Every Gynecologist Should Know About Perimenopause.* Clin Obstet Gynecol, 2020. **63**(4): p. 720-734.
42. Rybo, G., J. Leman, and E. Tibblin, *Epidemiology of menstrual blood loss,* in *Mechanisms of Menstrual Bleeding,* D.T. Baird and E.A. Mitchell, Editors. 1985, Raven Press New York: Edinburgh. p. 181-193.

43. Azlan, A., et al., *Endometrial inflammasome activation accompanies menstruation and may have implications for systemic inflammatory events of the menstrual cycle.* Hum Reprod, 2020. **35**(6): p. 1363-1376.

44. Critchley, H.O.D., et al., *Physiology of the Endometrium and Regulation of Menstruation.* Physiol Rev, 2020. **100**(3): p. 1149-1179.

45. Lethaby, A., K. Duckitt, and C. Farquhar, *Non-steroidal anti-inflammatory drugs for heavy menstrual bleeding.* Cochrane Database Syst Rev, 2013(1): p. Cd000400.

46. Rezk, M., A. Masood, and R. Dawood, *Perimenopausal bleeding: Patterns, pathology, response to progestins and clinical outcome.* J Obstet Gynaecol, 2015. **35**(5): p. 517-21.

47. Hale, G.E., et al., *Quantitative measurements of menstrual blood loss in ovulatory and anovulatory cycles in middle- and late-reproductive age and the menopausal transition.* Obstetrics & Gynecology, 2010. **115**(2 Pt 1): p. 249-56.

48. Whitaker, L. and H.O. Critchley, *Abnormal uterine bleeding.* Best Pract Res Clin Obstet Gynaecol, 2016. **34**: p. 54-65.

49. Borzutzky, C. and J. Jaffray, *Diagnosis and Management of Heavy Menstrual Bleeding and Bleeding Disorders in Adolescents.* JAMA Pediatr, 2020. **174**(2): p. 186-194.

50. Yang, Q., et al., *Comprehensive Review of Uterine Fibroids: Developmental Origin, Pathogenesis, and Treatment.* Endocr Rev, 2022. **43**(4): p. 678-719.

51. Ulin, M., et al., *Uterine fibroids in menopause and perimenopause.* Menopause, 2020. **27**(2): p. 238-242.

52. Yu, O., et al., *A US population-based study of uterine fibroid diagnosis incidence, trends, and prevalence: 2005 through 2014.* Am J Obstet Gynecol, 2018. **219**(6): p. 591.e1-591.e8.

53. Reis, F.M., E. Bloise, and T.M. Ortiga-Carvalho, *Hormones and pathogenesis of uterine fibroids.* Best Pract Res Clin Obstet Gynaecol, 2016. **34**: p. 13-24.

54. Giuliani, E., S. As-Sanie, and E.E. Marsh, *Epidemiology and management of uterine fibroids.* Int J Gynaecol Obstet, 2020. **149**(1): p. 3-9.

55. Haas, D., et al., *Endometriosis: a premenopausal disease? Age pattern in 42,079 patients with endometriosis.* Arch Gynecol Obstet, 2012. **286**(3): p. 667-70.

56. Jiang, L., et al., *Inflammation and endometriosis.* Front Biosci (Landmark Ed), 2016. **21**(5): p. 941-8.

57. Wei, Y., et al., *Autonomic nervous system and inflammation interaction in endometriosis-associated pain.* J Neuroinflammation, 2020. **17**(1): p. 80.

58. Parazzini, F., et al., *Epidemiology of endometriosis and its comorbidities.* Eur J Obstet Gynecol Reprod Biol, 2017. **209**: p. 3-7.

59. Lonsdorf, N., Butler, V., Brown, M., *A Woman's Best Medicine: Health, Happiness, and Long Life through Maharishi Ayur-Veda.* 1995, USA: TARCHER JEREMY PUBL.

60. Moieni, M., et al., *Exploring the role of gratitude and support-giving on inflammatory outcomes.* Emotion, 2019. **19**(6): p. 939-949.

61. Karns, C.M., W.E. Moore, 3rd, and U. Mayr, *The Cultivation of Pure Altruism via Gratitude: A Functional MRI Study of Change with Gratitude Practice.* Front Hum Neurosci, 2017. **11**: p. 599.

62. Moreno-Frías, C., N. Figueroa-Vega, and J.M. Malacara, *Relationship of sleep alterations with perimenopausal and postmenopausal symptoms.* Menopause, 2014. **21**(9): p. 1017-1022 10.1097/GME.0000000000000206.

63. Baker, F.C., et al., *Sleep and Sleep Disorders in the Menopausal Transition.* Sleep Med Clin, 2018. **13**(3): p. 443-456.

64. Kabat, G.C., et al., *The association of sleep duration and quality with all-cause and cause-specific mortality in the Women's Health Initiative.* Sleep Med, 2018. **50**: p. 48-54.

65. Kravitz, H.M., et al., *Sleep Trajectories Before and After the Final Menstrual Period in The Study of Women's Health Across the Nation (SWAN).* Curr Sleep Med Rep, 2017. **3**(3): p. 235-250.

66. Freeman, E.W., et al., *Poor sleep in relation to natural menopause: a population-based 14-year follow-up of midlife women.* Menopause, 2015. **22**(7): p. 719-26.

67. Lampio, L., et al., *Predictors of sleep disturbance in menopausal transition.* Maturitas, 2016. **94**: p. 137-142.

68. Shaver, J.L. and N.F. Woods, *Sleep and menopause: a narrative review.* Menopause, 2015. **22**(8): p. 899-915.

69. Xu, H., et al., *Are hot flashes associated with sleep disturbance during midlife? Results from the STRIDE cohort study.* Maturitas, 2012. **71**(1): p. 34-8.

70. Bromberger, J.T., et al., *Depressive symptoms during the menopausal transition: the Study of Women's Health Across the Nation (SWAN).* J Affect Disord, 2007. **103**(1-3): p. 267-72.

71. Zhou, Q., et al., *Investigation of the relationship between hot flashes, sweating and sleep quality in perimenopausal and postmenopausal women: the mediating effect of anxiety and depression.* BMC Womens Health, 2021. **21**(1): p. 293.

72. de Zambotti, M., et al., *Menstrual cycle-related variation in autonomic nervous system functioning in women in the early menopausal transition with and without insomnia disorder.* Psychoneuroendocrinology, 2017. **75**: p. 44-51.

73. Slopien, R., et al., *Disturbances of sleep continuity in women during the menopausal transition.* Psychiatr Pol, 2015. **49**(3): p. 615-23.

74. Cintron, D., et al., *Efficacy of menopausal hormone therapy on sleep quality: systematic review and meta-analysis.* Endocrine, 2017. **55**(3): p. 702-711.

75. Mirer, A.G., et al., *Sleep-disordered breathing and the menopausal transition among participants in the Sleep in Midlife Women Study.* Menopause, 2017. **24**(2): p. 157-162.

76. Adekolu, O. and A. Zinchuk, *Sleep Deficiency in Obstructive Sleep Apnea.* Clin Chest Med, 2022. **43**(2): p. 353-371.

77. Walker, M., *Why We Sleep.* 2018, Harlow, England: Penguin books.

78. Sexton, C.E., et al., *Connections Between Insomnia and Cognitive Aging.* Neurosci Bull, 2020. **36**(1): p. 77-84.

79. Scheyer, O., et al., *Female Sex and Alzheimer's Risk: The Menopause Connection.* J Prev Alzheimers Dis, 2018. **5**(4): p. 225-230.

80. Mosconi, L., *The XX Brain.* Vol. 1. 2020, USA: AVERY.

81. Mosconi, L., et al., *Increased Alzheimer's risk during the menopause transition: A 3-year longitudinal brain imaging study.* PLoS One, 2018. **13**(12): p. e0207885.

82. Iliff, J.J., et al., *A paravascular pathway facilitates CSF flow through the brain parenchyma and the clearance of interstitial solutes, including amyloid beta.* Sci Transl Med, 2012. **4**(147): p. 147ra111.

83. Bajda, J., N. Pitla, and V.R. Gorantla, *Bulat-Klarica-Oreskovic Hypothesis: A Comprehensive Review.* Cureus, 2023. **15**(9): p. e45821.

84. Krause, A.J., et al., *The Pain of Sleep Loss: A Brain Characterization in Humans.* J Neurosci, 2019. **39**(12): p. 2291-2300.

85. Saeedi, M. and A. Rashidy-Pour, *Association between chronic stress and Alzheimer's disease: Therapeutic effects of Saffron.* Biomed Pharmacother, 2021. **133**: p. 110995.

86. Carrion, V.G., et al., *Reduced hippocampal activity in youth with posttraumatic stress symptoms: an FMRI study.* J Pediatr Psychol, 2010. **35**(5): p. 559-69.

87. Kunimatsu, A., et al., *MRI findings in posttraumatic stress disorder.* J Magn Reson Imaging, 2020. **52**(2): p. 380-396.

88. Pertesi, S., et al., *Menopause, cognition and dementia - A review.* Post Reprod Health, 2019. **25**(4): p. 200-206.

89. Hung, S.Y. and W.M. Fu, *Drug candidates in clinical trials for Alzheimer's disease.* J Biomed Sci, 2017. **24**(1): p. 47.

90. McKenzie, J.A., et al., *Neuroinflammation as a Common Mechanism Associated with the Modifiable Risk Factors for Alzheimer's and Parkinson's Diseases.* Curr Aging Sci, 2017. **10**(3): p. 158-176.

91. Pistollato, F., et al., *Nutritional patterns associated with the maintenance of neurocognitive functions and the risk of dementia and Alzheimer's disease: A focus on human studies.* Pharmacol Res, 2018. **131**: p. 32-43.

92. Mayer, P., et al., *Autonomic Arousals as Surrogates for Cortical Arousals Caused by Respiratory Events: A Methodological Optimization Study in the Diagnosis of Sleep Breathing Disorders.* Nat Sci Sleep, 2019. **11**: p. 423-431.

93. Gabryelska, A. and P. Bialasiewicz, *Association between excessive daytime sleepiness, REM phenotype and severity of obstructive sleep apnea.* Sci Rep, 2020. **10**(1): p. 34.

94. Kravitz, H.M., R. Kazlauskaite, and H. Joffe, *Sleep, Health, and Metabolism in Midlife Women and Menopause: Food for Thought.* Obstet Gynecol Clin North Am, 2018. **45**(4): p. 679-694.

95. Aspevik, R.K. and O. Irtun, *[Complaints before and after cholecystectomy].* Tidsskr Nor Laegeforen, 2005. **125**(10): p. 1333-5.

96. Petroni, M.L., *Review article: gall-bladder motor function in obesity.* Aliment Pharmacol Ther, 2000. **14 Suppl 2**: p. 48-50.

97. Kucio, C., P. Besser, and K. Jonderko, *Gallbladder motor function in obese versus lean females.* Eur J Clin Nutr, 1988. **42**(2): p. 121-4.

98. Wang, H.H., et al., *New insights into the molecular mechanisms underlying effects of estrogen on cholesterol gallstone formation.* Biochim Biophys Acta, 2009. **1791**(11): p. 1037-47.

99. de Bari, O., et al., *Cholesterol cholelithiasis in pregnant women: pathogenesis, prevention and treatment.* Ann Hepatol, 2014. **13**(6): p. 728-45.

100. Sieron, D., et al., *The effect of chronic estrogen application on bile and gallstone composition in women with cholelithiasis.* Minerva Endocrinol, 2016. **41**(1): p. 19-27.

101. Honore, L.H., *Increased incidence of symptomatic cholesterol cholelithiasis in perimenopausal women receiving estrogen replacement therapy: a retrospective study.* J Reprod Med, 1980. **25**(4): p. 187-90.

102. Liu, X., et al., *Cholestasis-induced bile acid elevates estrogen level via farnesoid X receptor-mediated suppression of the estrogen sulfotransferase SULT1E1.* J Biol Chem, 2018. **293**(33): p. 12759-12769.

103. Sang, J.H., et al., *Correlations between metabolic syndrome, serologic factors, and gallstones.* J Phys Ther Sci, 2016. **28**(8): p. 2337-41.

104. Saklayen, M.G., *The Global Epidemic of the Metabolic Syndrome.* Curr Hypertens Rep, 2018. **20**(2): p. 12.

105. Pichetshote, N. and M. Pimentel, *An Approach to the Patient With Chronic Undiagnosed Abdominal Pain.* Am J Gastroenterol, 2019. **114**(5): p. 726-732.

106. Kashyap, P., et al., *Critical appraisal of the SIBO hypothesis and breath testing: A clinical practice update endorsed by the European society of neurogastroenterology and motility (ESNM) and the American neurogastroenterology and motility society (ANMS).* Neurogastroenterol Motil, 2024. **36**(6): p. e14817.

107. Ghoshal, U.C., R. Shukla, and U. Ghoshal, *Small Intestinal Bacterial Overgrowth and Irritable Bowel Syndrome: A Bridge between Functional Organic Dichotomy.* Gut Liver, 2017. **11**(2): p. 196-208.

108. Quigley, E.M.M., *The Spectrum of Small Intestinal Bacterial Overgrowth (SIBO).* Curr Gastroenterol Rep, 2019. **21**(1): p. 3.

109. Rezaie, A., et al., *Hydrogen and Methane-Based Breath Testing in Gastrointestinal Disorders: The North American Consensus.* Am J Gastroenterol, 2017. **112**(5): p. 775-784.

110. Chedid, V., et al., *Herbal therapy is equivalent to rifaximin for the treatment of small intestinal bacterial overgrowth.* Glob Adv Health Med, 2014. **3**(3): p. 16-24.

111. Barrett Mueller, K., et al., *Estrogen receptor inhibits mineralocorticoid receptor transcriptional regulatory function.* Endocrinology, 2014. **155**(11): p. 4461-72.

112. Lovick, T.A., et al., *A specific profile of luteal phase progesterone is associated with the development of premenstrual symptoms.* Psychoneuroendocrinology, 2017. **75**: p. 83-90.

113. Stachenfeld, N.S. and H.S. Taylor, *Effects of estrogen and progesterone administration on extracellular fluid.* J Appl Physiol (1985), 2004. **96**(3): p. 1011-8.

114. Giersch, G.E.W., et al., *Estrogen to Progesterone Ratio and Fluid Regulatory Responses to Varying Degrees and Methods of Dehydration.* Front Sports Act Living, 2021. **3**: p. 722305.

115. Janaki, K.L., et al., *Profile of Breast Diseases in Post Pubertal Women Assessed By Clinical Breast Examination - A Community Based Study in Rural Pondicherry.* J Clin Diagn Res, 2016. **10**(2): p. Pc07-11.

116. Koçoğlu, D., et al., *Mastalgia and associated factors: a cross-sectional study.* Agri, 2017. **29**(3): p. 100-108.

117. Altıntas, Y. and M. Bayrak, *Evaluation of 1294 Female Patients with Breast Pain: A Retrospective Study.* Adv Ther, 2018. **35**(9): p. 1411-1419.

118. Gong, C., et al., *A double-blind randomized controlled trial of toremifen therapy for mastalgia.* Arch Surg, 2006. **141**(1): p. 43-7.

119. Wisbey, J.R., et al., *Natural history of breast pain.* Lancet, 1983. **2**(8351): p. 672-4.

120. Brkić, M., et al., *THE ROLE OF E2/P RATIO IN THE ETIOLOGY OF FIBRO-CYSTIC BREAST DISEASE, MASTALGIA AND MASTODYNIA.* Acta Clin Croat, 2018. **57**(4): p. 756-761.

121. Martin, V.T., et al., *Perimenopause and Menopause Are Associated With High Frequency Headache in Women With Migraine: Results of the American Migraine Prevalence and Prevention Study.* Headache, 2016. **56**(2): p. 292-305.

122. Todd, C., A.M. Lagman-Bartolome, and C. Lay, *Women and Migraine: the Role of Hormones.* Curr Neurol Neurosci Rep, 2018. **18**(7): p. 42.

123. Allshouse, A., J. Pavlovic, and N. Santoro, *Menstrual Cycle Hormone Changes Associated with Reproductive Aging and How They May Relate to Symptoms.* Obstet Gynecol Clin North Am, 2018. **45**(4): p. 613-628.

124. Mulhall, S., R. Andel, and K.J. Anstey, *Variation in symptoms of depression and anxiety in midlife women by menopausal status.* Maturitas, 2018. **108**: p. 7-12.

125. Flores-Ramos, M., et al., *Evaluation of trait and state anxiety levels in a group of peri- and postmenopausal women.* Women Health, 2018. **58**(3): p. 305-319.

126. Vickers-Willis, R., *Navigating Midlife: Women Becoming Themselves.* 2022: Allen & Unwin Australia.

127. Usall, J., et al., *Suicide ideation across reproductive life cycle of women. Results from a European epidemiological study.* J Affect Disord, 2009. **116**(1-2): p. 144-7.

128. de Kruif, M., A.T. Spijker, and M.L. Molendijk, *Depression during the perimenopause: A meta-analysis.* J Affect Disord, 2016. **206**: p. 174-180.

129. Almeida, O.P., et al., *Depressive symptoms in midlife: the role of reproductive stage.* Menopause, 2016. **23**(6): p. 669-75.

130. Villa, A., et al., *Estrogens, Neuroinflammation, and Neurodegeneration.* Endocrine reviews, 2016. **37**(4): p. 372-402.

131. Cui, J., Y. Shen, and R. Li, *Estrogen synthesis and signaling pathways during aging: from periphery to brain.* Trends in molecular medicine, 2013. **19**(3): p. 197-209.

132. Lanza di Scalea, T. and T. Pearlstein, *Premenstrual Dysphoric Disorder.* Med Clin North Am, 2019. **103**(4): p. 613-628.

133. Jahanfar, S., M.S. Lye, and I.S. Krishnarajah, *The heritability of premenstrual syndrome.* Twin Res Hum Genet, 2011. **14**(5): p. 433-6.

134. Hashim, M.S., et al., *Premenstrual Syndrome Is Associated with Dietary and Lifestyle Behaviors among University Students: A Cross-Sectional Study from Sharjah, UAE.* Nutrients, 2019. **11**(8).

135. Roomruangwong, C., et al., *Lowered Plasma Steady-State Levels of Progesterone Combined With Declining Progesterone Levels During the Luteal Phase Predict Peri-Menstrual Syndrome and Its Major Subdomains.* Front Psychol, 2019. **10**: p. 2446.

136. Yen, J.Y., et al., *Estrogen levels, emotion regulation, and emotional symptoms of women with premenstrual dysphoric disorder: The moderating effect of estrogen receptor 1alpha polymorphism.* Prog Neuropsychopharmacol Biol Psychiatry, 2018. **82**: p. 216-223.

137. Imai, A., et al., *Premenstrual syndrome: management and pathophysiology.* Clin Exp Obstet Gynecol, 2015. **42**(2): p. 123-8.

138. Thomas, H.N., R. Hess, and R.C. Thurston, *Correlates of Sexual Activity and Satisfaction in Midlife and Older Women.* Ann Fam Med, 2015. **13**(4): p. 336-42.

139. Parish, S.J. and S.R. Hahn, *Hypoactive Sexual Desire Disorder: A Review of Epidemiology, Biopsychology, Diagnosis, and Treatment.* Sex Med Rev, 2016. **4**(2): p. 103-120.

140. Dennerstein, L., E. Dudley, and H. Burger, *Are changes in sexual functioning during midlife due to aging or menopause?* Fertility & Sterility, 2001. **76**(3): p. 456-60.

141. Gracia, C.R., et al., *Predictors of decreased libido in women during the late reproductive years.[see comment].* Menopause, 2004. **11**(2): p. 144-50.

142. Santoro, N., et al., *Correlates of circulating androgens in mid-life women: the study of women's health across the nation.* Journal of Clinical Endocrinology & Metabolism, 2005. **90**(8): p. 4836-45.

143. Davis, S.R., et al., *Testosterone enhances estradiol's effects on postmenopausal bone density and sexuality.* Maturitas, 1995. **21**(3): p. 227-36.

144. Goldstein, I., et al., *Hypoactive Sexual Desire Disorder: International Society for the Study of Women's Sexual Health (ISSWSH) Expert Consensus Panel Review.* Mayo Clin Proc, 2017. **92**(1): p. 114-128.

145. Hevesi, K., et al., *Different Characteristics of the Female Sexual Function Index in a Sample of Sexually Active and Inactive Women.* J Sex Med, 2017. **14**(9): p. 1133-1141.

146. Wiegel, M., C. Meston, and R. Rosen, *The female sexual function index (FSFI): cross-validation and development of clinical cutoff scores.* J Sex Marital Ther, 2005. **31**(1): p. 1-20.

147. Moen, P., *It's about time - Couples and Careers*, ed. P. Moen. 2003, New York: ILR Press, Cornell University Press.

148. Shitomi-Jones, L.M., et al., *Exploration of first onsets of mania, schizophrenia spectrum disorders and major depressive disorder in perimenopause.* Nature Mental Health, 2024: p. 1-8.

149. Caruso, S., et al., *Improvement of Low Sexual Desire Due to Antiandrogenic Combined Oral Contraceptives After Switching to an Oral Contraceptive Containing 17beta-Estradiol.* J Womens Health (Larchmt), 2017. **26**(7): p. 728-734.

150. Ciaplinskiene, L., et al., *The effect of a drospirenone-containing combined oral contraceptive on female sexual function: a prospective randomised study.* Eur J Contracept Reprod Health Care, 2016. **21**(5): p. 395-400.

151. Ishtiak-Ahmed, K., et al., *Midlife Forgetfulness and Risk of Dementia in Old Age: Results from the Danish Working Environment Cohort Study.* Dement Geriatr Cogn Disord, 2019. **47**(4-6): p. 264-273.

152. Guedj, A., et al., *Gut microbiota shape 'inflamm-ageing' cytokines and account for age-dependent decline in DNA damage repair.* Gut, 2020. **69**(6): p. 1064-1075.

153. Köhler, C.A., et al., *The Gut-Brain Axis, Including the Microbiome, Leaky Gut and Bacterial Translocation: Mechanisms and Pathophysiological Role in Alzheimer's Disease.* Curr Pharm Des, 2016. **22**(40): p. 6152-6166.

154. Margolis, K.G., J.F. Cryan, and E.A. Mayer, *The Microbiota-Gut-Brain Axis: From Motility to Mood.* Gastroenterology, 2021. **160**(5): p. 1486-1501.

155. Mayer, E.A., K. Nance, and S. Chen, *The Gut-Brain Axis.* Annu Rev Med, 2022. **73**: p. 439-453.

156. Marx, W., et al., *Nutritional psychiatry: the present state of the evidence.* Proc Nutr Soc, 2017. **76**(4): p. 427-436.

157. Rea, K., T.G. Dinan, and J.F. Cryan, *Gut Microbiota: A Perspective for Psychiatrists.* Neuropsychobiology, 2019: p. 1-13.

158. Arab, A., et al., *The association between diet and mood: A systematic review of current literature.* Psychiatry Res, 2019. **271**: p. 428-437.

159. Rutsch, A., J.B. Kantsjö, and F. Ronchi, *The Gut-Brain Axis: How Microbiota and Host Inflammasome Influence Brain Physiology and Pathology.* Front Immunol, 2020. **11**: p. 604179.

160. Hou, X., et al., *GABAergic System in Stress: Implications of GABAergic Neuron Subpopulations and the Gut-Vagus-Brain Pathway.* Neural Plast, 2020. **2020**: p. 8858415.

161. Fasano, A., *All disease begins in the (leaky) gut: role of zonulin-mediated gut permeability in the pathogenesis of some chronic inflammatory diseases.* F1000Res, 2020. **9**.

162. Camilleri, M., *Leaky gut: mechanisms, measurement and clinical implications in humans.* Gut, 2019. **68**(8): p. 1516-1526.

163. Srikantha, P. and M.H. Mohajeri, *The Possible Role of the Microbiota-Gut-Brain-Axis in Autism Spectrum Disorder.* Int J Mol Sci, 2019. **20**(9).

164. Morris, G., et al., *Leaky brain in neurological and psychiatric disorders: Drivers and consequences.* Aust N Z J Psychiatry, 2018. **52**(10): p. 924-948.

165. Maes, M., et al., *Breakdown of the Paracellular Tight and Adherens Junctions in the Gut and Blood Brain Barrier and Damage to the Vascular Barrier in Patients with Deficit Schizophrenia.* Neurotox Res, 2019. **36**(2): p. 306-322.

166. Wardlaw, J.M., C. Smith, and M. Dichgans, *Small vessel disease: mechanisms and clinical implications.* Lancet Neurol, 2019. **18**(7): p. 684-696.

167. Wardlaw, J.M., M.C. Valdes Hernandez, and S. Munoz-Maniega, *What are white matter hyperintensities made of? Relevance to vascular cognitive impairment.* J Am Heart Assoc, 2015. **4**(6): p. 001140.

168. Ross, D.E., et al., *Man Versus Machine Part 2: Comparison of Radiologists' Interpretations and NeuroQuant Measures of Brain Asymmetry and Progressive Atrophy in Patients With Traumatic Brain Injury.* J Neuropsychiatry Clin Neurosci, 2015. **27**(2): p. 147-52.

169. Fraga-Silva, T.F.C., et al., *Gliotoxin Aggravates Experimental Autoimmune Encephalomyelitis by Triggering Neuroinflammation.* Toxins (Basel), 2019. **11**(8).

170. Harding, C.F., et al., *Mold inhalation causes innate immune activation, neural, cognitive and emotional dysfunction.* Brain Behav Immun, 2019.

171. Robbins, C.A., et al., *Health effects of mycotoxins in indoor air: a critical review.* Appl Occup Environ Hyg, 2000. **15**(10): p. 773-84.

172. Gulpers, B.J.A., et al., *Anxiety as a Risk Factor for Cognitive Decline: A 12-Year Follow-Up Cohort Study.* Am J Geriatr Psychiatry, 2019. **27**(1): p. 42-52.

173. Christian, K.M., H. Song, and G.L. Ming, *Functions and dysfunctions of adult hippocampal neurogenesis.* Annu Rev Neurosci, 2014. **37**: p. 243-62.

174. Peng, L. and M.A. Bonaguidi, *Function and Dysfunction of Adult Hippocampal Neurogenesis in Regeneration and Disease.* Am J Pathol, 2018. **188**(1): p. 23-28.

175. Fedoce, A.D.G., et al., *The role of oxidative stress in anxiety disorder: cause or consequence?* Free Radic Res, 2018. **52**(7): p. 737-750.

176. Cobley, J.N., M.L. Fiorello, and D.M. Bailey, *13 reasons why the brain is susceptible to oxidative stress.* Redox Biol, 2018. **15**: p. 490-503.

177. Gulpers, B., et al., *Anxiety as a Predictor for Cognitive Decline and Dementia: A Systematic Review and Meta-Analysis.* Am J Geriatr Psychiatry, 2016. **24**(10): p. 823-42.

178. Hale, G.E., et al., *Cyclicity of breast tenderness and night-time vasomotor symptoms in mid-life women: information collected using the Daily Perimenopause Diary.* Climacteric, 2003. **6**(2): p. 128-39.

179. Freeman, E.W., et al., *Symptom reports from a cohort of African American and white women in the late reproductive years.* Menopause, 2001. **8**(1): p. 33-42.

180. Williams, R.E., et al., *Frequency and severity of vasomotor symptoms among peri- and postmenopausal women in the United States.* Climacteric, 2008. **11**(1): p. 32-43.

181. Thurston, R.C., *Vasomotor symptoms: natural history, physiology, and links with cardiovascular health.* Climacteric, 2018. **21**(2): p. 96-100.

182. Vermeulen, R.F.M., et al., *Impact of risk-reducing salpingo-oophorectomy in premenopausal women.* Climacteric, 2017. **20**(3): p. 212-221.

183. Hall, E., et al., *Effects of bilateral salpingo-oophorectomy on menopausal symptoms and sexual functioning among women with a BRCA1 or BRCA2 mutation.* Gynecol Oncol, 2019. **152**(1): p. 145-150.

184. Rance, N.E., et al., *Modulation of body temperature and LH secretion by hypothalamic KNDy (kisspeptin, neurokinin B and dynorphin) neurons: a novel hypothesis on the mechanism of hot flushes.* Front Neuroendocrinol, 2013. **34**(3): p. 211-27.

185. Oakley, A.E., et al., *kappa Agonists as a novel therapy for menopausal hot flashes.* Menopause, 2015. **22**(12): p. 1328-34.

186. Neal-Perry, G., et al., *Safety of Fezolinetant for Vasomotor Symptoms Associated With Menopause: A Randomized Controlled Trial.* Obstet Gynecol, 2023. **141**(4): p. 737-747.

187. Johnson, K.A., et al., *Efficacy and Safety of Fezolinetant in Moderate to Severe Vasomotor Symptoms Associated With Menopause: A Phase 3 RCT.* J Clin Endocrinol Metab, 2023. **108**(8): p. 1981-1997.

188. Prior, J.C., et al., *Determination of luteal phase length by quantitative basal temperature methods: validation against the mid-cycle LH peak.* Clinical & Investigative Medicine - Medecine Clinique et Experimentale, 1990. **13**(3): p. 123-31.

189. Prior, J.C., *Progesterone for treatment of symptomatic menopausal women.* Climacteric, 2018. **21**(4): p. 358-365.

190. Reed, S.D., et al., *Self-reported menopausal symptoms in a racially diverse population and soy food consumption.* Maturitas, 2013. **75**(2): p. 152-8.

191. Crandall, C.J., et al., *Genetic Variation and Hot Flashes: A Systematic Review.* J Clin Endocrinol Metab, 2020. **105**(12): p. e4907-57.

192. Saccomani, S., et al., *Does obesity increase the risk of hot flashes among midlife women?: a population-based study.* Menopause, 2017. **24**(9): p. 1065-1070.

193. Hyde Riley, E., et al., *Differential association of modifiable health behaviors with hot flashes in perimenopausal and postmenopausal women.* J Gen Intern Med, 2004. **19**(7): p. 740-6.

194. Schilling, C., et al., *Current alcohol use, hormone levels, and hot flashes in midlife women.* Fertil Steril, 2007. **87**(6): p. 1483-6.

195. Freeman, E.W., et al., *Hot flashes in the late reproductive years: risk factors for Africa American and Caucasian women.* J Womens Health Gend Based Med, 2001. **10**(1): p. 67-76.

196. Chen, W.Y., et al., *Moderate alcohol consumption during adult life, drinking patterns, and breast cancer risk.* Jama, 2011. **306**(17): p. 1884-90.

197. Shield, K.D., I. Soerjomataram, and J. Rehm, *Alcohol Use and Breast Cancer: A Critical Review.* Alcohol Clin Exp Res, 2016. **40**(6): p. 1166-81.

198. Mahabir, S., et al., *Effects of low-to-moderate alcohol supplementation on urinary estrogen metabolites in postmenopausal women in a controlled feeding study.* Cancer Med, 2017. **6**(10): p. 2419-2423.

199. Hartman, T.J., et al., *Alcohol Consumption and Urinary Estrogens and Estrogen Metabolites in Premenopausal Women.* Horm Cancer, 2016. **7**(1): p. 65-74.

200. Goel, S., A. Sharma, and A. Garg, *Effect of Alcohol Consumption on Cardiovascular Health.* Curr Cardiol Rep, 2018. **20**(4): p. 19.

201. Mitchell, E.S. and N.F. Woods, *Cognitive symptoms during the menopausal transition and early postmenopause.* Climacteric, 2011. **14**(2): p. 252-61.

202. Sood, R., et al., *Association of mindfulness and stress with menopausal symptoms in midlife women.* Climacteric, 2019: p. 1-6.

203. Bauld, R. and R.F. Brown, *Stress, psychological distress, psychosocial factors, menopause symptoms and physical health in women.* Maturitas, 2009. **62**(2): p. 160-5.

204. Yao, B.C., et al., *Chronic stress: a critical risk factor for atherosclerosis.* J Int Med Res, 2019. **47**(4): p. 1429-1440.

205. van Ravenswaaij-Arts, C.M., et al., *Heart rate variability.* Ann Intern Med, 1993. **118**(6): p. 436-47.

206. Muka, T., et al., *Association of Vasomotor and Other Menopausal Symptoms with Risk of Cardiovascular Disease: A Systematic Review and Meta-Analysis.* PLoS One, 2016. **11**(6): p. e0157417.

207. Gast, G.C., et al., *Vasomotor menopausal symptoms are associated with increased risk of coronary heart disease.* Menopause, 2011. **18**(2): p. 146-51.

208. Hautamaki, H., et al., *Cardiovascular autonomic responsiveness in postmenopausal women with and without hot flushes.* Maturitas, 2011. **68**(4): p. 368-73.

209. Li, J., X. Yi, and J. Ai, *Broaden Horizons: The Advancement of Interstitial Cystitis/Bladder Pain Syndrome.* Int J Mol Sci, 2022. **23**(23).

210. Wen, C., L. Xie, and C. Hu, *Roles of mesenchymal stem cells and exosomes in interstitial cystitis/bladder pain syndrome.* J Cell Mol Med, 2022. **26**(3): p. 624-635.

211. Afrin, L.B., et al., *Successful mast-cell-targeted treatment of chronic dyspareunia, vaginitis, and dysfunctional uterine bleeding.* J Obstet Gynaecol, 2019. **39**(5): p. 664-669.

212. Theoharides, T.C., I. Tsilioni, and H. Ren, *Recent advances in our understanding of mast cell activation - or should it be mast cell mediator disorders?* Expert Rev Clin Immunol, 2019. **15**(6): p. 639-656.

213. Karlamangla, A.S., S.M. Burnett-Bowie, and C.J. Crandall, *Bone Health During the Menopause Transition and Beyond.* Obstet Gynecol Clin North Am, 2018. **45**(4): p. 695-708.

214. Prior, J.C., *Progesterone for the prevention and treatment of osteoporosis in women.* Climacteric, 2018. **21**(4): p. 366-374.
215. Chin, K.Y., *The Relationship between Follicle-stimulating Hormone and Bone Health: Alternative Explanation for Bone Loss beyond Oestrogen?* Int J Med Sci, 2018. **15**(12): p. 1373-1383.
216. Engin, A., *Obesity-associated Breast Cancer: Analysis of risk factors.* Adv Exp Med Biol, 2017. **960**: p. 571-606.
217. Martens, P.J., et al., *Vitamin D's Effect on Immune Function.* Nutrients, 2020. **12**(5).
218. Sebtain, A., et al., *Subclinical Hypothyroidism in Perimenopausal Abnormal Uterine Bleeding Patients.* Cureus, 2022. **14**(2): p. e21839.
219. Goyal, G., et al., *Subclinical Hypothyroidism and Associated Cardiovascular Risk Factor in Perimenopausal Females.* J Midlife Health, 2020. **11**(1): p. 6-11.
220. Kim, Y., et al., *The Prevalence of Thyroid Dysfunction in Korean Women Undergoing Routine Health Screening: A Cross-Sectional Study.* Thyroid, 2022. **32**(7): p. 819-827.
221. Frank-Raue, K. and F. Raue, *Thyroid Dysfunction in Periand Postmenopausal Women-Cumulative Risks.* Dtsch Arztebl Int, 2023. **120**(18): p. 311-316.
222. Kjaergaard, A.D., et al., *Thyroid function, sex hormones and sexual function: a Mendelian randomization study.* Eur J Epidemiol, 2021. **36**(3): p. 335-344.
223. Vanderpump, M.P.J., *The epidemiology of thyroid disease.* British Medical Bulletin, 2011. **99**(1): p. 39-51.
224. Moulton, V.R., *Sex Hormones in Acquired Immunity and Autoimmune Disease.* Front Immunol, 2018. **9**: p. 2279.
225. Trenti, A., et al., *Estrogen, Angiogenesis, Immunity and Cell Metabolism: Solving the Puzzle.* Int J Mol Sci, 2018. **19**(3).
226. Hu, X., et al., *Cancer Risk in Hashimoto's Thyroiditis: a Systematic Review and Meta-Analysis.* Front Endocrinol (Lausanne), 2022. **13**: p. 937871.
227. Pearce, E.N. and M.B. Zimmermann, *The Prevention of Iodine Deficiency: A History.* Thyroid, 2023. **33**(2): p. 143-149.
228. Thorburn, A.N., L. Macia, and C.R. Mackay, *Diet, metabolites, and "western-lifestyle" inflammatory diseases.* Immunity, 2014. **40**(6): p. 833-42.
229. Helander, H.F. and L. Fändriks, *Surface area of the digestive tract - revisited.* Scand J Gastroenterol, 2014. **49**(6): p. 681-9.
230. Schoultz, I. and V. Keita Å, *The Intestinal Barrier and Current Techniques for the Assessment of Gut Permeability.* Cells, 2020. **9**(8).
231. Tilg, H., et al., *The intestinal microbiota fuelling metabolic inflammation.* Nat Rev Immunol, 2020. **20**(1): p. 40-54.
232. Malesza, I.J., et al., *High-Fat, Western-Style Diet, Systemic Inflammation, and Gut Microbiota: A Narrative Review.* Cells, 2021. **10**(11).
233. Minihane, A.M., et al., *Low-grade inflammation, diet composition and health: current research evidence and its translation.* Br J Nutr, 2015. **114**(7): p. 999-1012.

234. Imhann, F., et al., *Proton pump inhibitors affect the gut microbiome.* Gut, 2016. **65**(5): p. 740-8.

235. Minalyan, A., et al., *The Gastric and Intestinal Microbiome: Role of Proton Pump Inhibitors.* Curr Gastroenterol Rep, 2017. **19**(8): p. 42.

236. Martinsen, T.C., R. Fossmark, and H.L. Waldum, *The Phylogeny and Biological Function of Gastric Juice-Microbiological Consequences of Removing Gastric Acid.* Int J Mol Sci, 2019. **20**(23).

237. Untersmayr, E. and E. Jensen-Jarolim, *The role of protein digestibility and antacids on food allergy outcomes.* J Allergy Clin Immunol, 2008. **121**(6): p. 1301-8; quiz 1309-10.

238. Ayazi, S., et al., *Measurement of gastric pH in ambulatory esophageal pH monitoring.* Surg Endosc, 2009. **23**(9): p. 1968-73.

239. Yago, M.R., et al., *The use of betaine HCl to enhance dasatinib absorption in healthy volunteers with rabeprazole-induced hypochlorhydria.* Aaps j, 2014. **16**(6): p. 1358-65.

240. Dandona, P., A. Aljada, and A. Bandyopadhyay, *Inflammation: the link between insulin resistance, obesity and diabetes.* Trends Immunol, 2004. **25**(1): p. 4-7.

241. De Felice, F.G. and S.T. Ferreira, *Inflammation, defective insulin signaling, and mitochondrial dysfunction as common molecular denominators connecting type 2 diabetes to Alzheimer disease.* Diabetes, 2014. **63**(7): p. 2262-72.

242. Jha, J.C., et al., *A causal link between oxidative stress and inflammation in cardiovascular and renal complications of diabetes.* Clin Sci (Lond), 2018. **132**(16): p. 1811-1836.

243. Ormazabal, V., et al., *Association between insulin resistance and the development of cardiovascular disease.* Cardiovasc Diabetol, 2018. **17**(1): p. 122.

244. Razmjou, S., et al., *Body composition, cardiometabolic risk factors, physical activity, and inflammatory markers in premenopausal women after a 10-year follow-up: a MONET study.* Menopause, 2018. **25**(1): p. 89-97.

245. Wojciechowska, J., et al., *Diabetes and Cancer: a Review of Current Knowledge.* Exp Clin Endocrinol Diabetes, 2016. **124**(5): p. 263-75.

246. Dabrowski, M., et al., *Risk factors for cancer development in type 2 diabetes: A retrospective case-control study.* BMC Cancer, 2016. **16**(1): p. 785.

247. Unamuno, X., et al., *Adipokine dysregulation and adipose tissue inflammation in human obesity.* Eur J Clin Invest, 2018. **48**(9): p. e12997.

248. DiNicolantonio, J.J. and J.H. O'Keefe, *Good Fats versus Bad Fats: A Comparison of Fatty Acids in the Promotion of Insulin Resistance, Inflammation, and Obesity.* Mo Med, 2017. **114**(4): p. 303-307.

249. Garbossa, S.G. and F. Folli, *Vitamin D, sub-inflammation and insulin resistance. A window on a potential role for the interaction between bone and glucose metabolism.* Rev Endocr Metab Disord, 2017. **18**(2): p. 243-258.

250. Lammers, K.M., et al., *Gliadin Induces Neutrophil Migration via Engagement of the Formyl Peptide Receptor, FPR1.* PLoS One, 2015. **10**(9): p. e0138338.

251. Lammers, K.M., et al., *Gliadin induces an increase in intestinal permeability and zonulin release by binding to the chemokine receptor CXCR3.* Gastroenterology, 2008. **135**(1): p. 194-204.e3.
252. Valitutti, F. and A. Fasano, *Breaking Down Barriers: How Understanding Celiac Disease Pathogenesis Informed the Development of Novel Treatments.* Dig Dis Sci, 2019. **64**(7): p. 1748-1758.
253. Shin, W. and H.J. Kim, *Intestinal barrier dysfunction orchestrates the onset of inflammatory host-microbiome cross-talk in a human gut inflammation-on-a-chip.* Proc Natl Acad Sci U S A, 2018. **115**(45): p. E10539-e10547.
254. Farshchi, M.K., et al., *A Viewpoint on the Leaky Gut Syndrome to Treat Allergic Asthma: A Novel Opinion.* J Evid Based Complementary Altern Med, 2017. **22**(3): p. 378-380.
255. Mu, Q., et al., *Leaky Gut As a Danger Signal for Autoimmune Diseases.* Front Immunol, 2017. **8**: p. 598.
256. Riccio, P. and R. Rossano, *Undigested Food and Gut Microbiota May Cooperate in the Pathogenesis of Neuroinflammatory Diseases: A Matter of Barriers and a Proposal on the Origin of Organ Specificity.* Nutrients, 2019. **11**(11).
257. Volta, U., et al., *Non-coeliac gluten/wheat sensitivity: advances in knowledge and relevant questions.* Expert Rev Gastroenterol Hepatol, 2017. **11**(1): p. 9-18.
258. Tortora, R., et al., *Metabolic syndrome in patients with coeliac disease on a gluten-free diet.* Aliment Pharmacol Ther, 2015. **41**(4): p. 352-9.
259. Samsel, A. and S. Seneff, *Glyphosate, pathways to modern diseases II: Celiac sprue and gluten intolerance.* Interdiscip Toxicol, 2013. **6**(4): p. 159-84.
260. Potter, M., et al., *Incidence and prevalence of self-reported non-coeliac wheat sensitivity and gluten avoidance in Australia.* Med J Aust, 2020. **212**(3): p. 126-131.
261. Motta, E.V.S., K. Raymann, and N.A. Moran, *Glyphosate perturbs the gut microbiota of honey bees.* Proc Natl Acad Sci U S A, 2018. **115**(41): p. 10305-10310.
262. Davoren, M.J. and R.H. Schiestl, *Glyphosate-based herbicides and cancer risk: a post-IARC decision review of potential mechanisms, policy and avenues of research.* Carcinogenesis, 2018. **39**(10): p. 1207-1215.
263. Rueda-Ruzafa, L., et al., *Gut microbiota and neurological effects of glyphosate.* Neurotoxicology, 2019. **75**: p. 1-8.
264. Barnett, J.A. and D.L. Gibson, *Separating the Empirical Wheat From the Pseudoscientific Chaff: A Critical Review of the Literature Surrounding Glyphosate, Dysbiosis and Wheat-Sensitivity.* Front Microbiol, 2020. **11**: p. 556729.
265. Winstone, J.K., et al., *Correction: Glyphosate infiltrates the brain and increases pro-inflammatory cytokine TNFα: implications for neurodegenerative disorders.* J Neuroinflammation, 2024. **21**(1): p. 20.
266. Meiers, J., et al., *Lectin antagonists in infection, immunity, and inflammation.* Curr Opin Chem Biol, 2019. **53**: p. 51-67.
267. Frosh, A., et al., *Effect of a dairy diet on nasopharyngeal mucus secretion.* Laryngoscope, 2019. **129**(1): p. 13-17.

268. Anthoni, S., et al., *Milk protein IgG and IgA: the association with milk-induced gastro-intestinal symptoms in adults.* World J Gastroenterol, 2009. **15**(39): p. 4915-8.

269. Brooke-Taylor, S., et al., *Systematic Review of the Gastrointestinal Effects of A1 Compared with A2 β-Casein.* Adv Nutr, 2017. **8**(5): p. 739-748.

270. Jeong, H., Y.S. Park, and S.S. Yoon, *A2 milk consumption and its health benefits: an update.* Food Sci Biotechnol, 2024. **33**(3): p. 491-503.

271. Platel, K. and K. Srinivasan, *Digestive stimulant action of spices: a myth or reality?* Indian J Med Res, 2004. **119**(5): p. 167-79.

272. Prakash, U.N. and K. Srinivasan, *Enhanced intestinal uptake of iron, zinc and calcium in rats fed pungent spice principles--piperine, capsaicin and ginger (Zingiber officinale).* J Trace Elem Med Biol, 2013. **27**(3): p. 184-90.

273. Van Hecke, T., et al., *Long-Chain n-3 PUFA Content and n-6/n-3 PUFA Ratio in Mammal, Poultry, and Fish Muscles Largely Explain Differential Protein and Lipid Oxidation Profiles Following In Vitro Gastrointestinal Digestion.* Mol Nutr Food Res, 2019. **63**(22): p. e1900404.

274. Mugnai, C., et al., *The effects of husbandry system on the grass intake and egg nutritive characteristics of laying hens.* J Sci Food Agric, 2014. **94**(3): p. 459-67.

275. Jaček, M., et al., *Effect of Food with Low Enrichment of N-3 Fatty Acids in a Two-Month Diet on the Fatty Acid Content in the Plasma and Erythrocytes and on Cardiovascular Risk Markers in Healthy Young Men.* Nutrients, 2020. **12**(8).

276. Fruet, A.P.B., et al., *Oxidative stability of beef from steers finished exclusively with concentrate, supplemented, or on legume-grass pasture.* Meat Sci, 2018. **145**: p. 121-126.

277. Carabante, K.M., et al., *Consumer Acceptance, Emotional Response, and Purchase Intent of Rib-Eye Steaks from Grass-Fed Steers, and Effects of Health Benefit Information on Consumer Perception.* J Food Sci, 2018. **83**(10): p. 2560-2570.

278. Rhodes, C.J., *The imperative for regenerative agriculture.* Sci Prog, 2017. **100**(1): p. 80-129.

279. Jordon, M.W., et al., *Can Regenerative Agriculture increase national soil carbon stocks? Simulated country-scale adoption of reduced tillage, cover cropping, and ley-arable integration using RothC.* Sci Total Environ, 2022. **825**: p. 153955.

280. Turesky, R.J., *Mechanistic Evidence for Red Meat and Processed Meat Intake and Cancer Risk: A Follow-up on the International Agency for Research on Cancer Evaluation of 2015.* Chimia (Aarau), 2018. **72**(10): p. 718-724.

281. Zhong, V.W., et al., *Associations of Processed Meat, Unprocessed Red Meat, Poultry, or Fish Intake With Incident Cardiovascular Disease and All-Cause Mortality.* JAMA Intern Med, 2020. **180**(4): p. 503-512.

282. Uribarri, J., et al., *Dietary advanced glycation end products and their role in health and disease.* Adv Nutr, 2015. **6**(4): p. 461-73.

283. Uribarri, J., et al., *Advanced glycation end products in foods and a practical guide to their reduction in the diet.* J Am Diet Assoc, 2010. **110**(6): p. 911-16.e12.

284. Gill, V., et al., *Advanced Glycation End Products (AGEs) May Be a Striking Link Between Modern Diet and Health.* Biomolecules, 2019. **9**(12).

285. Kheirouri, S., M. Alizadeh, and V. Maleki, *Zinc against advanced glycation end products.* Clin Exp Pharmacol Physiol, 2018. **45**(6): p. 491-498.

286. Urban, L.E., et al., *Temporal trends in fast-food restaurant energy, sodium, saturated fat, and trans fat content, United States, 1996-2013.* Prev Chronic Dis, 2014. **11**: p. E229.

287. DiMarco, D.M., et al., *Intake of up to 3 Eggs/Day Increases HDL Cholesterol and Plasma Choline While Plasma Trimethylamine-N-oxide is Unchanged in a Healthy Population.* Lipids, 2017. **52**(3): p. 255-263.

288. Liguori, I., et al., *Oxidative stress, aging, and diseases.* Clin Interv Aging, 2018. **13**: p. 757-772.

289. Nowson, C. and S. O'Connell, *Protein Requirements and Recommendations for Older People: A Review.* Nutrients, 2015. **7**(8): p. 6874-99.

290. Leonard, B.E., *Inflammation and depression: a causal or coincidental link to the pathophysiology?* Acta Neuropsychiatr, 2018. **30**(1): p. 1-16.

291. Sanders, V.M. and R.H. Straub, *Norepinephrine, the beta-adrenergic receptor, and immunity.* Brain Behav Immun, 2002. **16**(4): p. 290-332.

292. Umamaheswaran, S., et al., *Stress, inflammation, and eicosanoids: an emerging perspective.* Cancer Metastasis Rev, 2018. **37**(2-3): p. 203-211.

293. Rohleder, N., *Stress and inflammation - The need to address the gap in the transition between acute and chronic stress effects.* Psychoneuroendocrinology, 2019. **105**: p. 164-171.

294. Breit, S., et al., *Vagus Nerve as Modulator of the Brain-Gut Axis in Psychiatric and Inflammatory Disorders.* Front Psychiatry, 2018. **9**: p. 44.

295. Telles, S., et al., *Alternate-Nostril Yoga Breathing Reduced Blood Pressure While Increasing Performance in a Vigilance Test.* Med Sci Monit Basic Res, 2017. **23**: p. 392-398.

296. Telles, S., et al., *Changes in Shape and Size Discrimination and State Anxiety After Alternate-Nostril Yoga Breathing and Breath Awareness in One Session Each.* Med Sci Monit Basic Res, 2019. **25**: p. 121-127.

297. Liu, Y., et al., *The effectiveness of diaphragmatic breathing relaxation training for improving sleep quality among nursing staff during the COVID-19 outbreak: a before and after study.* Sleep medicine, 2021. **78**: p. 8-14.

298. Tobe, M. and S. Saito, *Analogy between classical Yoga/Zen breathing and modern clinical respiratory therapy.* Journal of anesthesia, 2020. **34**(6): p. 944-949.

299. Zou, L., et al., *A Systematic Review and Meta-Analysis Baduanjin Qigong for Health Benefits: Randomized Controlled Trials.* Evid Based Complement Alternat Med, 2017. **2017**: p. 4548706.

300. Hendriks, T., J. de Jong, and H. Cramer, *The Effects of Yoga on Positive Mental Health Among Healthy Adults: A Systematic Review and Meta-Analysis.* J Altern Complement Med, 2017. **23**(7): p. 505-517.

301. Thongtipmak, S., et al., *Immediate Effects and Acceptability of an Application-Based Stretching Exercise Incorporating Deep Slow Breathing for Neck Pain Self-management.* Healthcare informatics research, 2020. **26**(1): p. 50-60.

302. Wongwilairat, K., et al., *Muscle stretching with deep and slow breathing patterns: a pilot study for therapeutic development.* J Complement Integr Med, 2018. **16**(2).

303. Yamanaka, Y., *Basic concepts and unique features of human circadian rhythms: implications for human health.* Nutr Rev, 2020. **78**(12 Suppl 2): p. 91-96.

304. Kyeong, S., et al., *Effects of gratitude meditation on neural network functional connectivity and brain-heart coupling.* Sci Rep, 2017. **7**(1): p. 5058.

305. Rao, A., et al., *Prayer or spiritual healing as adjuncts to conventional care: a cross sectional analysis of prevalence and characteristics of use among women.* BMJ Open, 2015. **5**(6): p. e007345.

306. Deepak, K.K., *Meditation induces physical relaxation and enhances cognition: A perplexing paradox.* Prog Brain Res, 2019. **244**: p. 85-99.

307. Cavalieri, E.L. and E.G. Rogan, *Depurinating estrogen-DNA adducts in the etiology and prevention of breast and other human cancers.* Future Oncology, 2010. **6**(1): p. 75-91.

308. Yager, J.D., *Mechanisms of estrogen carcinogenesis: The role of E2/E1-quinone metabolites suggests new approaches to preventive intervention--A review.* Steroids, 2015. **99**(Pt A): p. 56-60.

309. Santen, R.J., W. Yue, and J.P. Wang, *Estrogen metabolites and breast cancer.* Steroids, 2015. **99**(Pt A): p. 61-6.

310. Liew, S.C. and E.D. Gupta, *Methylenetetrahydrofolate reductase (MTHFR) C677T polymorphism: epidemiology, metabolism and the associated diseases.* Eur J Med Genet, 2015. **58**(1): p. 1-10.

311. von Wedel-Parlow, M., P. Wolte, and H.J. Galla, *Regulation of major efflux transporters under inflammatory conditions at the blood-brain barrier in vitro.* J Neurochem, 2009. **111**(1): p. 111-8.

312. Jetter, A. and G.A. Kullak-Ublick, *Drugs and hepatic transporters: A review.* Pharmacol Res, 2019: p. 104234.

313. Hale, G.E., et al., *A double-blind randomized study on the effects of red clover isoflavones on the endometrium.* Menopause, 2001. **8**(5): p. 338-346.

314. Hale, G.E., et al., *Isoflavone supplementation and endothalial function in menopausal women.* Clinical Endocrinology, 2002. **56**: p. 693-701.

315. Bijlsma, N. and M.M. Cohen, *Expert clinician's perspectives on environmental medicine and toxicant assessment in clinical practice.* Environ Health Prev Med, 2018. **23**(1): p. 19.

316. Monneret, C., *What is an endocrine disruptor?* C R Biol, 2017. **340**(9-10): p. 403-405.

317. Shafei, A., et al., *The molecular mechanisms of action of the endocrine disrupting chemical bisphenol A in the development of cancer.* Gene, 2018. **647**: p. 235-243.

318. Schug, T.T., et al., *Minireview: Endocrine Disruptors: Past Lessons and Future Directions.* Mol Endocrinol, 2016. **30**(8): p. 833-47.

319. Aylward, L.L., et al., *Relationships of chemical concentrations in maternal and cord blood: a review of available data.* J Toxicol Environ Health B Crit Rev, 2014. **17**(3): p. 175-203.

320. Nomiri, S., et al., *A mini review of bisphenol A (BPA) effects on cancer-related cellular signaling pathways.* Environ Sci Pollut Res Int, 2019. **26**(9): p. 8459-8467.

321. Gross, L. and L.S. Birnbaum, *Regulating toxic chemicals for public and environmental health.* PLoS Biol, 2017. **15**(12): p. e2004814.

322. Wielsoe, M., P. Kern, and E.C. Bonefeld-Jorgensen, *Serum levels of environmental pollutants is a risk factor for breast cancer in Inuit: a case control study.* Environ Health, 2017. **16**(1): p. 56.

323. Teixeira, D., et al., *Inflammatory and cardiometabolic risk on obesity: role of environmental xenoestrogens.* J Clin Endocrinol Metab, 2015. **100**(5): p. 1792-801.

324. Jafari, T., et al., *The association between mercury levels and autism spectrum disorders: A systematic review and meta-analysis.* J Trace Elem Med Biol, 2017. **44**: p. 289-297.

325. Rooney, J.P., *The retention time of inorganic mercury in the brain--a systematic review of the evidence.* Toxicol Appl Pharmacol, 2014. **274**(3): p. 425-35.

326. Bondy, S.C., *Prolonged exposure to low levels of aluminum leads to changes associated with brain aging and neurodegeneration.* Toxicology, 2014. **315**: p. 1-7.

327. Stellaard, F. and D. Lütjohann, *Dynamics of the enterohepatic circulation of bile acids in healthy humans.* Am J Physiol Gastrointest Liver Physiol, 2021. **321**(1): p. G55-g66.

328. Parida, S. and D. Sharma, *The Microbiome-Estrogen Connection and Breast Cancer Risk.* Cells, 2019. **8**(12).

329. Zhou, X., et al., *Enterohepatic circulation of glucuronide metabolites of drugs in dog.* Pharmacol Res Perspect, 2019. **7**(4): p. e00502.

330. Yaghjyan, L., et al., *Associations of gut microbiome with endogenous estrogen levels in healthy postmenopausal women.* Cancer Causes Control, 2023. **34**(10): p. 873-881.

331. Wu, Z., et al., *Associations of Circulating Estrogens and Estrogen Metabolites with Fecal and Oral Microbiome in Postmenopausal Women in the Ghana Breast Health Study.* Microbiol Spectr, 2023. **11**(4): p. e0157223.

332. Thibaut, M.M. and L.B. Bindels, *Crosstalk between bile acid-activated receptors and microbiome in entero-hepatic inflammation.* Trends Mol Med, 2022. **28**(3): p. 223-236.

333. Zheng, Z., J.L. Fang, and P. Lazarus, *Glucuronidation: an important mechanism for detoxification of benzo[a]pyrene metabolites in aerodigestive tract tissues.* Drug Metab Dispos, 2002. **30**(4): p. 397-403.

334. Awolade, P., et al., *Therapeutic significance of β-glucuronidase activity and its inhibitors: A review.* Eur J Med Chem, 2020. **187**: p. 111921.

335. Baker, J.M., L. Al-Nakkash, and M.M. Herbst-Kralovetz, *Estrogen-gut microbiome axis: Physiological and clinical implications.* Maturitas, 2017. **103**: p. 45-53.
336. Dwivedi, C., et al., *Effect of calcium glucarate on beta-glucuronidase activity and glucarate content of certain vegetables and fruits.* Biochem Med Metab Biol, 1990. **43**(2): p. 83-92.
337. Sugimoto, K., et al., *Dietary Bamboo Charcoal Decreased Visceral Adipose Tissue Weight by Enhancing Fecal Lipid Excretions in Mice with High-Fat Diet-Induced Obesity.* Prev Nutr Food Sci, 2023. **28**(3): p. 246-254.
338. Zellner, T., et al., *The Use of Activated Charcoal to Treat Intoxications.* Dtsch Arztebl Int, 2019. **116**(18): p. 311-317.
339. Bhatti, S.A., et al., *Comparative efficacy of Bentonite clay, activated charcoal and Trichosporon mycotoxinivorans in regulating the feed-to-tissue transfer of mycotoxins.* J Sci Food Agric, 2018. **98**(3): p. 884-890.
340. Melchior, C., et al., *Efficacy of antibiotherapy for treating flatus incontinence associated with small intestinal bacterial overgrowth: A pilot randomized trial.* PLoS One, 2017. **12**(8): p. e0180835.
341. Fuchs, C.D. and M. Trauner, *Role of bile acids and their receptors in gastrointestinal and hepatic pathophysiology.* Nat Rev Gastroenterol Hepatol, 2022. **19**(7): p. 432-450.
342. Ismail, A., L. Kennedy, and H. Francis, *Sex-Dependent Differences in Cholestasis: Why Estrogen Signaling May Be a Key Pathophysiological Driver.* Am J Pathol, 2023. **193**(10): p. 1355-1362.
343. Shaik, F.A., et al., *Bitter taste receptors: Extraoral roles in pathophysiology.* Int J Biochem Cell Biol, 2016. **77**(Pt B): p. 197-204.
344. McMullen, M.K., J.M. Whitehouse, and A. Towell, *Bitters: Time for a New Paradigm.* Evid Based Complement Alternat Med, 2015. **2015**: p. 670504.
345. Wang, J., et al., *Assessing the Effects of Ginger Extract on Polyphenol Profiles and the Subsequent Impact on the Fecal Microbiota by Simulating Digestion and Fermentation In Vitro.* Nutrients, 2020. **12**(10).
346. Anh, N.H., et al., *Ginger on Human Health: A Comprehensive Systematic Review of 109 Randomized Controlled Trials.* Nutrients, 2020. **12**(1).
347. Seo, S.H., F. Fang, and I. Kang, *Ginger (Zingiber officinale) Attenuates Obesity and Adipose Tissue Remodeling in High-Fat Diet-Fed C57BL/6 Mice.* Int J Environ Res Public Health, 2021. **18**(2).
348. Hofmann, T., et al., *Modulation of detoxification enzymes by watercress: in vitro and in vivo investigations in human peripheral blood cells.* Eur J Nutr, 2009. **48**(8): p. 483-91.
349. Khanum, F., et al., *Effects of feeding fresh garlic and garlic oil on detoxifying enzymes and micronuclei formation in rats treated with azoxymethane.* Int J Vitam Nutr Res, 1998. **68**(3): p. 208-13.
350. Wettasinghe, M., et al., *Phase II enzyme-inducing and antioxidant activities of*

beetroot (Beta vulgaris L.) extracts from phenotypes of different pigmentation. J Agric Food Chem, 2002. **50**(23): p. 6704-9.

351. Krajka-Kuźniak, V., et al., *Beetroot juice protects against N-nitrosodiethylamine-induced liver injury in rats.* Food Chem Toxicol, 2012. **50**(6): p. 2027-33.

352. Jeffery, E.H. and K.E. Stewart, *Upregulation of quinone reductase by glucosinolate hydrolysis products from dietary broccoli.* Methods Enzymol, 2004. **382**: p. 457-69.

353. Fernández-Iglesias, A., et al., *Combination of grape seed proanthocyanidin extract and docosahexaenoic acid-rich oil increases the hepatic detoxification by GST mediated GSH conjugation in a lipidic postprandial state.* Food Chem, 2014. **165**: p. 14-20.

354. Rodríguez-Ramiro, I., et al., *Procyanidin B2 induces Nrf2 translocation and glutathione S-transferase P1 expression via ERKs and p38-MAPK pathways and protect human colonic cells against oxidative stress.* Eur J Nutr, 2012. **51**(7): p. 881-92.

355. Satoh, T., et al., *Inhibitory Effects of Eight Green Tea Catechins on Cytochrome P450 1A2, 2C9, 2D6, and 3A4 Activities.* J Pharm Pharm Sci, 2016. **19**(2): p. 188-97.

356. Wu, A.H., et al., *Tea and circulating estrogen levels in postmenopausal Chinese women in Singapore.* Carcinogenesis, 2005. **26**(5): p. 976-80.

357. Faria, A., et al., *Pomegranate juice effects on cytochrome P450S expression: in vivo studies.* J Med Food, 2007. **10**(4): p. 643-9.

358. Basten, G.P., Y. Bao, and G. Williamson, *Sulforaphane and its glutathione conjugate but not sulforaphane nitrile induce UDP-glucuronosyl transferase (UGT1A1) and glutathione transferase (GSTA1) in cultured cells.* Carcinogenesis, 2002. **23**(8): p. 1399-404.

359. Yoxall, V., et al., *Modulation of hepatic cytochromes P450 and phase II enzymes by dietary doses of sulforaphane in rats: Implications for its chemopreventive activity.* Int J Cancer, 2005. **117**(3): p. 356-62.

360. Skarpanska-Stejnborn, A., et al., *The influence of supplementation with artichoke (Cynara scolymus L.) extract on selected redox parameters in rowers.* Int J Sport Nutr Exerc Metab, 2008. **18**(3): p. 313-27.

361. Kotronoulas, A., et al., *Dose-dependent metabolic disposition of hydroxytyrosol and formation of mercapturates in rats.* Pharmacol Res, 2013. **77**: p. 47-56.

362. Visioli, F., et al., *Olive phenolics increase glutathione levels in healthy volunteers.* J Agric Food Chem, 2009. **57**(5): p. 1793-6.

363. Alp, H., et al., *Effects of sulforophane and curcumin on oxidative stress created by acute malathion toxicity in rats.* Eur Rev Med Pharmacol Sci, 2012. **16 Suppl 3**: p. 144-8.

364. Guo, Y., et al., *Arsenic methylation by an arsenite S-adenosylmethionine methyltransferase from Spirulina platensis.* J Environ Sci (China), 2016. **49**: p. 162-168.

365. Gupta, R. and S.J. Flora, *Protective value of Aloe vera against some toxic effects of arsenic in rats.* Phytother Res, 2005. **19**(1): p. 23-8.

366. Vrba, J., et al., *Identification of UDP-glucuronosyltransferases involved in the*

metabolism of silymarin flavonolignans. J Pharm Biomed Anal, 2020. **178**: p. 112972.

367. Soleimani, V., et al., *Safety and toxicity of silymarin, the major constituent of milk thistle extract: An updated review.* Phytother Res, 2019. **33**(6): p. 1627-1638.

368. Kiruthiga, P.V., et al., *Silymarin protection against major reactive oxygen species released by environmental toxins: exogenous H2O2 exposure in erythrocytes.* Basic Clin Pharmacol Toxicol, 2007. **100**(6): p. 414-9.

369. Alaca, N., et al., *Treatment with milk thistle extract (Silybum marianum), ursode-oxycholic acid, or their combination attenuates cholestatic liver injury in rats: Role of the hepatic stem cells.* Turk J Gastroenterol, 2017. **28**(6): p. 476-484.

370. Lii, C.K., et al., *Sulforaphane and alpha-lipoic acid upregulate the expression of the pi class of glutathione S-transferase through c-jun and Nrf2 activation.* J Nutr, 2010. **140**(5): p. 885-92.

371. Singh, B., et al., *Resveratrol inhibits estrogen-induced breast carcinogenesis through induction of NRF2-mediated protective pathways.* Carcinogenesis, 2014. **35**(8): p. 1872-80.

372. Parkin, D.R. and D. Malejka-Giganti, *Differences in the hepatic P450-dependent metabolism of estrogen and tamoxifen in response to treatment of rats with 3,3'-diindolylmethane and its parent compound indole-3-carbinol.* Cancer Detect Prev, 2004. **28**(1): p. 72-9.

373. Thomson, C.A., et al., *A randomized, placebo-controlled trial of diindolylmethane for breast cancer biomarker modulation in patients taking tamoxifen.* Breast Cancer Res Treat, 2017. **165**(1): p. 97-107.

374. Fanti, M., et al., *Time-Restricted Eating, Intermittent Fasting, and Fasting-Mimicking Diets in Weight Loss.* Curr Obes Rep, 2021. **10**(2): p. 70-80.

375. Longo, V.D. and S. Panda, *Fasting, Circadian Rhythms, and Time-Restricted Feeding in Healthy Lifespan.* Cell Metab, 2016. **23**(6): p. 1048-1059.

376. Elortegui Pascual, P., et al., *A meta-analysis comparing the effectiveness of alternate day fasting, the 5:2 diet, and time-restricted eating for weight loss.* Obesity (Silver Spring), 2023. **31 Suppl 1**(Suppl 1): p. 9-21.

377. Cienfuegos, S., et al., *Time restricted eating for the prevention of type 2 diabetes.* J Physiol, 2022. **600**(5): p. 1253-1264.

378. Mishra, S., et al., *Time-Restricted Eating and Its Metabolic Benefits.* J Clin Med, 2023. **12**(22).

379. Barati, M., A. Ghahremani, and H. Namdar Ahmadabad, *Intermittent fasting: A promising dietary intervention for autoimmune diseases.* Autoimmun Rev, 2023. **22**(10): p. 103408.

380. Henmi, H., et al., *Effects of ascorbic acid supplementation on serum progesterone levels in patients with a luteal phase defect.* Fertil Steril, 2003. **80**(2): p. 459-61.

381. Miszkiel, G., et al., *Concentrations of catecholamines, ascorbic acid, progesterone and oxytocin in the corpora lutea of cyclic and pregnant cattle.* Reprod Nutr Dev, 1999. **39**(4): p. 509-16.

382. Griesinger, G., et al., *Ascorbic acid supplement during luteal phase in IVF.* J Assist Reprod Genet, 2002. **19**(4): p. 164-8.

383. Spoelstra-de Man, A.M.E., P.W.G. Elbers, and H.M. Oudemans-Van Straaten, *Vitamin C: should we supplement?* Curr Opin Crit Care, 2018. **24**(4): p. 248-255.

384. Paschalis, V., et al., *Low vitamin C values are linked with decreased physical performance and increased oxidative stress: reversal by vitamin C supplementation.* Eur J Nutr, 2016. **55**(1): p. 45-53.

385. Barreca, D., et al., *Flavanones: Citrus phytochemical with health-promoting properties.* Biofactors, 2017. **43**(4): p. 495-506.

386. Boyle, N.B., C. Lawton, and L. Dye, *The Effects of Magnesium Supplementation on Subjective Anxiety and Stress-A Systematic Review.* Nutrients, 2017. **9**(5).

387. Boyle, N.B., C.L. Lawton, and L. Dye, *The effects of magnesium supplementation on subjective anxiety.* Magnes Res, 2016. **29**(3): p. 120-125.

388. McCabe, D., et al., *The impact of essential fatty acid, B vitamins, vitamin C, magnesium and zinc supplementation on stress levels in women: a systematic review.* JBI Database System Rev Implement Rep, 2017. **15**(2): p. 402-453.

389. Wang, S.F., et al., *Acute restraint stress triggers progesterone withdrawal and endometrial breakdown and shedding through corticosterone stimulation in mouse menstrual-like model.* Reproduction, 2019. **157**(2): p. 149-161.

390. Lee, Y. and E.O. Im, *Stress and premenstrual symptoms among Korean women studying in the U.S. and South Korea: A longitudinal web-based study.* Women Health, 2017. **57**(6): p. 665-684.

391. Sampaio, C.V., M.G. Lima, and A.M. Ladeia, *Meditation, Health and Scientific Investigations: Review of the Literature.* J Relig Health, 2017. **56**(2): p. 411-427.

392. Zou, L., et al., *The Effect of Taichi Practice on Attenuating Bone Mineral Density Loss: A Systematic Review and Meta-Analysis of Randomized Controlled Trials.* Int J Environ Res Public Health, 2017. **14**(9).

393. Clark, I. and H.P. Landolt, *Coffee, caffeine, and sleep: A systematic review of epidemiological studies and randomized controlled trials.* Sleep Med Rev, 2017. **31**: p. 70-78.

394. Ooi, S.L., et al., *Vitex Agnus-Castus for the Treatment of Cyclic Mastalgia: A Systematic Review and Meta-Analysis.* J Womens Health (Larchmt), 2020. **29**(2): p. 262-278.

395. Mollazadeh, S., M. Mirghafourvand, and N.G. Abdollahi, *The effects of Vitex agnus-castus on menstrual bleeding: A systematic review and meta-analysis.* J Complement Integr Med, 2019.

396. Csupor, D., et al., *Vitex agnus-castus in premenstrual syndrome: A meta-analysis of double-blind randomised controlled trials.* Complement Ther Med, 2019. **47**: p. 102190.

397. Verkaik, S., et al., *The treatment of premenstrual syndrome with preparations of Vitex agnus castus: a systematic review and meta-analysis.* Am J Obstet Gynecol, 2017. **217**(2): p. 150-166.

398. Falahat, F., et al., *Efficacy of a Herbal Formulation Based on Foeniculum Vulgare in Oligo/Amenorrhea: A Randomized Clinical Trial.* Curr Drug Discov Technol, 2018.

399. Zeqiri, A., M. Dermaku-Sopjani, and M. Sopjani, *The mechanisms underlying the role of Vitex agnus-castus in mastalgia.* Bratisl Lek Listy, 2022. **123**(12): p. 913-918.

400. Męczekalski, B. and A. Czyżyk, *[Vitex Agnus Castus in the treatment of hyperprolactinemia and menstrual disorders - a case report].* Pol Merkur Lekarski, 2015. **39**(229): p. 43-6.

401. van Die, M.D., et al., *Vitex agnus-castus extracts for female reproductive disorders: a systematic review of clinical trials.* Planta Med, 2013. **79**(7): p. 562-75.

402. Ahangarpour, A., S.A. Najimi, and Y. Farbood, *Effects of Vitex agnus-castus fruit on sex hormones and antioxidant indices in a d-galactose-induced aging female mouse model.* J Chin Med Assoc, 2016. **79**(11): p. 589-596.

403. Matsui, M., et al., *Characterisation of the anti-inflammatory potential of Vitex trifolia L. (Labiatae), a multipurpose plant of the Pacific traditional medicine.* J Ethnopharmacol, 2009. **126**(3): p. 427-33.

404. Daniele, C., et al., *Vitex agnus castus: a systematic review of adverse events.* Drug Saf, 2005. **28**(4): p. 319-32.

405. Jewson, M., P. Purohit, and M.A. Lumsden, *Progesterone and abnormal uterine bleeding/menstrual disorders.* Best Pract Res Clin Obstet Gynaecol, 2020. **69**: p. 62-73.

406. Ford, O., et al., *Progesterone for premenstrual syndrome.* Cochrane Database Syst Rev, 2012. **2012**(3): p. Cd003415.

407. Hellberg, D., B. Claesson, and S. Nilsson, *Premenstrual tension: a placebo-controlled efficacy study with spironolactone and medroxyprogesterone acetate.* Int J Gynaecol Obstet, 1991. **34**(3): p. 243-8.

408. Maddox, P.R., et al., *A randomised controlled trial of medroxyprogesterone acetate in mastalgia.* Ann R Coll Surg Engl, 1990. **72**(2): p. 71-6.

409. Naheed, B., et al., *Non-contraceptive oestrogen-containing preparations for controlling symptoms of premenstrual syndrome.* Cochrane Database Syst Rev, 2017. **3**: p. Cd010503.

410. Asi, N., et al., *Progesterone vs. synthetic progestins and the risk of breast cancer: a systematic review and meta-analysis.* Syst Rev, 2016. **5**(1): p. 121.

411. Caufriez, A., et al., *Progesterone prevents sleep disturbances and modulates GH, TSH, and melatonin secretion in postmenopausal women.* J Clin Endocrinol Metab, 2011. **96**(4): p. E614-23.

412. Wren, B.G., et al., *Effect of sequential transdermal progesterone cream on endometrium, bleeding pattern, and plasma progesterone and salivary progesterone levels in postmenopausal women.* Climacteric, 2000. **3**(3): p. 155-60.

413. Wren, B.G., et al., *Transdermal progesterone and its effect on vasomotor symptoms, blood lipid levels, bone metabolic markers, moods, and quality of life for postmenopausal women.* Menopause, 2003. **10**(1): p. 13-8.

414. Stanczyk, F.Z., R.J. Paulson, and S. Roy, *Percutaneous administration of progesterone: blood levels and endometrial protection.* Menopause, 2005. **12**(2): p. 232-7.

415. Du, J.Y., et al., *Percutaneous progesterone delivery via cream or gel application in postmenopausal women: a randomized cross-over study of progesterone levels in serum, whole blood, saliva, and capillary blood.* Menopause, 2013. **20**(11): p. 1169-75.

416. Bofill Rodriguez, M., A. Lethaby, and C. Farquhar, *Non-steroidal anti-inflammatory drugs for heavy menstrual bleeding.* Cochrane Database Syst Rev, 2019. **9**(9): p. Cd000400.

417. Nikkhah, S., et al., *Effects of boron supplementation on the severity and duration of pain in primary dysmenorrhea.* Complement Ther Clin Pract, 2015. **21**(2): p. 79-83.

418. Maybin, J.A. and H.O. Critchley, *Medical management of heavy menstrual bleeding.* Womens Health (Lond), 2016. **12**(1): p. 27-34.

419. Minalt, N., C.D. Canela, and S. Marino, *Endometrial Ablation,* in *StatPearls.* 2024, StatPearls Publishing

Copyright © 2024, StatPearls Publishing LLC.: Treasure Island (FL) ineligible companies. Disclosure: Christinne Canela declares no relevant financial relationships with ineligible companies. Disclosure: Sarah Marino declares no relevant financial relationships with ineligible companies.

420. Emslie, E., et al., *Evaluation of Radiofrequency Endometrial Ablation: A 17-year Canadian Experience.* J Minim Invasive Gynecol, 2023. **30**(11): p. 905-911.

421. Katon, J.G., et al., *Trends in hysterectomy rates among women veterans in the US Department of Veterans Affairs.* Am J Obstet Gynecol, 2017. **217**(4): p. 428. e1-428.e11.

422. Wilson, L.F., N. Pandeya, and G.D. Mishra, *Hysterectomy trends in Australia, 2000-2001 to 2013-2014: joinpoint regression analysis.* Acta Obstet Gynecol Scand, 2017. **96**(10): p. 1170-1179.

423. Borahay, M.A., et al., *Estrogen Receptors and Signaling in Fibroids: Role in Pathobiology and Therapeutic Implications.* Reprod Sci, 2017. **24**(9): p. 1235-1244.

424. Borghini, R., et al., *Irritable Bowel Syndrome-Like Disorders in Endometriosis: Prevalence of Nickel Sensitivity and Effects of a Low-Nickel Diet. An Open-Label Pilot Study.* Nutrients, 2020. **12**(2).

425. Ciebiera, M., et al., *The Evolving Role of Natural Compounds in the Medical Treatment of Uterine Fibroids.* J Clin Med, 2020. **9**(5).

426. Stewart, J.K., *Uterine Artery Embolization for Uterine Fibroids: A Closer Look at Misperceptions and Challenges.* Tech Vasc Interv Radiol, 2021. **24**(1): p. 100725.

427. Ramdhan, R.C., M. Loukas, and R.S. Tubbs, *Anatomical complications of hysterectomy: A review.* Clin Anat, 2017. **30**(7): p. 946-952.

428. As-Sanie, S., et al., *Incidence and predictors of persistent pelvic pain following hysterectomy in women with chronic pelvic pain.* Am J Obstet Gynecol, 2021. **225**(5): p. 568.e1-568.e11.

429. Crocetto, F., et al., *Urinary Incontinence after Planned Cesarean Hysterectomy for Placenta Accreta.* Urol Int, 2021. **105**(11-12): p. 1099-1103.
430. Skorupska, K., et al., *Impact of Hysterectomy on Quality of Life, Urinary Incontinence, Sexual Functions and Urethral Length.* J Clin Med, 2021. **10**(16).
431. Maas, C.P., P.T.M. Weijenborg, and M.M. Ter Kuile, *The effect of hysterectomy on sexual functioning.* Annual Review of Sex Research, 2003. **14**: p. 83-113.
432. Dilbaz, B. and A. Aksan, *Premenstrual syndrome, a common but underrated entity: review of the clinical literature.* J Turk Ger Gynecol Assoc, 2021. **22**(2): p. 139-148.
433. Piette, P.C.M., *The pharmacodynamics and safety of progesterone.* Best Pract Res Clin Obstet Gynaecol, 2020. **69**: p. 13-29.
434. Stoddard, F.R., 2nd, et al., *Iodine alters gene expression in the MCF7 breast cancer cell line: evidence for an anti-estrogen effect of iodine.* International journal of medical sciences, 2008. **5**(4): p. 189-196.
435. Lasley, B.L., S. Crawford, and D.S. McConnell, *Adrenal androgens and the menopausal transition.* Obstet Gynecol Clin North Am, 2011. **38**(3): p. 467-75.
436. Serra, D., L.M. Almeida, and T.C.P. Dinis, *The Impact of Chronic Intestinal Inflammation on Brain Disorders: the Microbiota-Gut-Brain Axis.* Mol Neurobiol, 2019. **56**(10): p. 6941-6951.
437. Cryan, J.F., et al., *The Microbiota-Gut-Brain Axis.* Physiol Rev, 2019. **99**(4): p. 1877-2013.
438. Evrensel, A., B. Ünsalver, and M.E. Ceylan, *Neuroinflammation, Gut-Brain Axis and Depression.* Psychiatry Investig, 2020. **17**(1): p. 2-8.
439. Lozza-Fiacco, S., et al., *Baseline anxiety-sensitivity to estradiol fluctuations predicts anxiety symptom response to transdermal estradiol treatment in perimenopausal women - A randomized clinical trial.* Psychoneuroendocrinology, 2022. **143**: p. 105851.
440. Ono, D. and A. Yamanaka, *Hypothalamic regulation of the sleep/wake cycle.* Neurosci Res, 2017. **118**: p. 74-81.
441. Kim, J.H. and H.J. Yu, *The Effectiveness of Cognitive Behavioral Therapy on Depression and Sleep Problems for Climacteric Women: A Systematic Review and Meta-Analysis.* J Clin Med, 2024. **13**(2).
442. Janku, K., et al., *Block the light and sleep well: Evening blue light filtration as a part of cognitive behavioral therapy for insomnia.* Chronobiol Int, 2019: p. 1-12.
443. Ishitsuka, Y., Y. Kondo, and D. Kadowaki, *Toxicological Property of Acetaminophen: The Dark Side of a Safe Antipyretic/Analgesic Drug?* Biol Pharm Bull, 2020. **43**(2): p. 195-206.
444. Louvet, A., et al., *Acute Liver Injury With Therapeutic Doses of Acetaminophen: A Prospective Study.* Hepatology, 2021. **73**(5): p. 1945-1955.
445. Schormair, B., et al., *Genome-wide meta-analyses of restless legs syndrome yield insights into genetic architecture, disease biology and risk prediction.* Nat Genet, 2024. **56**(6): p. 1090-1099.

446. Nanayakkara, B., J. Di Michiel, and B.J. Yee, *Restless legs syndrome.* Aust J Gen Pract, 2023. **52**(9): p. 615-621.

447. Landolt, H.P., et al., *Zolpidem and sleep deprivation: different effect on EEG power spectra.* J Sleep Res, 2000. **9**(2): p. 175-83.

448. Choi, J.W., et al., *Use of Sedative-Hypnotics and Mortality: A Population-Based Retrospective Cohort Study.* J Clin Sleep Med, 2018. **14**(10): p. 1669-1677.

449. Parsaik, A.K., et al., *Mortality associated with anxiolytic and hypnotic drugs-A systematic review and meta-analysis.* Aust N Z J Psychiatry, 2016. **50**(6): p. 520-33.

450. Zarezadeh, M., et al., *Melatonin supplementation and pro-inflammatory mediators: a systematic review and meta-analysis of clinical trials.* Eur J Nutr, 2020. **59**(5): p. 1803-1813.

451. Golabchi, A., et al., *Melatonin improves quality and longevity of chronic neural recording.* Biomaterials, 2018. **180**: p. 225-239.

452. Jenwitheesuk, A., et al., *Melatonin regulates aging and neurodegeneration through energy metabolism, epigenetics, autophagy and circadian rhythm pathways.* Int J Mol Sci, 2014. **15**(9): p. 16848-84.

453. Mortezaee, K., et al., *Boosting immune system against cancer by melatonin: A mechanistic viewpoint.* Life Sci, 2019. **238**: p. 116960.

454. Yamadera, W., et al., *Glycine ingestion improves subjective sleep quality in human volunteers, correlating with polysomnographic changes.* Sleep and Biological Rhythms, 2007. **5**(2): p. 126-131.

455. Kawai, N., et al., *The sleep-promoting and hypothermic effects of glycine are mediated by NMDA receptors in the suprachiasmatic nucleus.* Neuropsychopharmacology, 2015. **40**(6): p. 1405-16.

456. Inagawa, K., et al., *Subjective effects of glycine ingestion before bedtime on sleep quality.* Sleep and Biological Rhythms, 2006. **4**(1): p. 75-77.

457. McCarty, M.F., J.H. O'Keefe, and J.J. DiNicolantonio, *Dietary Glycine Is Rate-Limiting for Glutathione Synthesis and May Have Broad Potential for Health Protection.* Ochsner J, 2018. **18**(1): p. 81-87.

458. Razak, M.A., et al., *Multifarious Beneficial Effect of Nonessential Amino Acid, Glycine: A Review.* Oxid Med Cell Longev, 2017. **2017**: p. 1716701.

459. Mah, J. and T. Pitre, *Oral magnesium supplementation for insomnia in older adults: a Systematic Review & Meta-Analysis.* BMC Complement Med Ther, 2021. **21**(1): p. 125.

460. Jakaria, M., et al., *Taurine and its analogs in neurological disorders: Focus on therapeutic potential and molecular mechanisms.* Redox Biol, 2019. **24**: p. 101223.

461. Nolan, B.J., B. Liang, and A.S. Cheung, *Efficacy of Micronized Progesterone for Sleep: A Systematic Review and Meta-analysis of Randomized Controlled Trial Data.* J Clin Endocrinol Metab, 2021. **106**(4): p. 942-951.

462. Ramos, A.R., A.G. Wheaton, and D.A. Johnson, *Sleep Deprivation, Sleep Disorders, and Chronic Disease.* Prev Chronic Dis, 2023. **20**: p. E77.

463. de Zambotti, M., et al., *The Sleep of the Ring: Comparison of the ŌURA Sleep Tracker Against Polysomnography.* Behav Sleep Med, 2019. **17**(2): p. 124-136.

464. Berryhill, S., et al., *Effect of wearables on sleep in healthy individuals: a randomized crossover trial and validation study.* J Clin Sleep Med, 2020. **16**(5): p. 775-783.

465. Savolainen-Peltonen, H., et al., *Use of postmenopausal hormone therapy and risk of Alzheimer's disease in Finland: nationwide case-control study.* Bmj, 2019. **364**: p. l665.

466. Baik, S.H., F. Baye, and C.J. McDonald, *Use of menopausal hormone therapy beyond age 65 years and its effects on women's health outcomes by types, routes, and doses.* Menopause, 2024. **31**(5): p. 363-371.

467. Nerattini, M., et al., *Systematic review and meta-analysis of the effects of menopause hormone therapy on risk of Alzheimer's disease and dementia.* Front Aging Neurosci, 2023. **15**: p. 1260427.

468. Chiu, H.Y., et al., *Cholesterol Levels, Hormone Replacement Therapy, and Incident Dementia among Older Adult Women.* Nutrients, 2023. **15**(20).

469. Steventon, J.J., et al., *Menopause age, reproductive span and hormone therapy duration predict the volume of medial temporal lobe brain structures in postmenopausal women.* Psychoneuroendocrinology, 2023. **158**: p. 106393.

470. Yuk, J.S., J.S. Lee, and J.H. Park, *Menopausal hormone therapy and risk of dementia: health insurance database in South Korea-based retrospective cohort study.* Front Aging Neurosci, 2023. **15**: p. 1213481.

471. Hao, W., et al., *Age at menopause and all-cause and cause-specific dementia: a prospective analysis of the UK Biobank cohort.* Hum Reprod, 2023. **38**(9): p. 1746-1754.

472. Wood Alexander, M., et al., *Associations Between Age at Menopause, Vascular Risk, and 3-Year Cognitive Change in the Canadian Longitudinal Study on Aging.* Neurology, 2024. **102**(9): p. e209298.

473. Rocca, W.A., K. Kantarci, and S.S. Faubion, *Risks and benefits of hormone therapy after menopause for cognitive decline and dementia: A conceptual review.* Maturitas, 2024. **184**: p. 108003.

474. Youwakim, J. and H. Girouard, *Inflammation: A Mediator Between Hypertension and Neurodegenerative Diseases.* Am J Hypertens, 2021. **34**(10): p. 1014-1030.

475. Rajan, K.B., et al., *Blood pressure and risk of incident Alzheimer's disease dementia by antihypertensive medications and APOE ε4 allele.* Ann Neurol, 2018. **83**(5): p. 935-944.

476. Grandl, G. and C. Wolfrum, *Hemostasis, endothelial stress, inflammation, and the metabolic syndrome.* Semin Immunopathol, 2018. **40**(2): p. 215-224.

477. Xiao, L. and D.G. Harrison, *Inflammation in Hypertension.* Can J Cardiol, 2020. **36**(5): p. 635-647.

478. Bello-Chavolla, O.Y., et al., *Pathophysiological Mechanisms Linking Type 2 Diabetes and Dementia: Review of Evidence from Clinical, Translational and Epidemiological Research.* Curr Diabetes Rev, 2019. **15**(6): p. 456-470.

479. Cooper, C., et al., *Modifiable predictors of dementia in mild cognitive impairment: a systematic review and meta-analysis.* Am J Psychiatry, 2015. **172**(4): p. 323-34.

480. Washington, P.M., S. Villapol, and M.P. Burns, *Polypathology and dementia after brain trauma: Does brain injury trigger distinct neurodegenerative diseases, or should they be classified together as traumatic encephalopathy?* Exp Neurol, 2016. **275 Pt 3**(0 3): p. 381-388.

481. Chen, X., et al., *Omega-3 polyunsaturated fatty acid attenuates traumatic brain injury-induced neuronal apoptosis by inducing autophagy through the upregulation of SIRT1-mediated deacetylation of Beclin-1.* J Neuroinflammation, 2018. **15**(1): p. 310.

482. Siblerud, R., et al., *A Hypothesis and Evidence That Mercury May be an Etiological Factor in Alzheimer's Disease.* Int J Environ Res Public Health, 2019. **16**(24).

483. Guzzi, G., et al., *Dental amalgam and mercury levels in autopsy tissues: food for thought.* Am J Forensic Med Pathol, 2006. **27**(1): p. 42-5.

484. Omura, Y., et al., *Significant mercury deposits in internal organs following the removal of dental amalgam, & development of pre-cancer on the gingiva and the sides of the tongue and their represented organs as a result of inadvertent exposure to strong curing light (used to solidify synthetic dental filling material) & effective treatment: a clinical case report, along with organ representation areas for each tooth.* Acupunct Electrother Res, 1996. **21**(2): p. 133-60.

485. Morris, M.C., et al., *Association of Seafood Consumption, Brain Mercury Level, and APOE ε4 Status With Brain Neuropathology in Older Adults.* Jama, 2016. **315**(5): p. 489-97.

486. Mueller, A., et al., *Individual and combined effects of mycotoxins from typical indoor moulds.* Toxicol In Vitro, 2013. **27**(6): p. 1970-8.

487. Daly, B., et al., *Evidence summary: the relationship between oral health and dementia.* Br Dent J, 2018. **223**(11): p. 846-853.

488. Jung, H.J., et al., *Chronic rhinosinusitis and progression of cognitive impairment in dementia.* Eur Ann Otorhinolaryngol Head Neck Dis, 2020.

489. Chung, S.D., et al., *Dementia is associated with chronic rhinosinusitis: a population-based case-controlled study.* Am J Rhinol Allergy, 2015. **29**(1): p. 44-7.

490. Bairey Merz, C.N., et al., *Knowledge, Attitudes, and Beliefs Regarding Cardiovascular Disease in Women: The Women's Heart Alliance.* J Am Coll Cardiol, 2017. **70**(2): p. 123-132.

491. Colpani, V., et al., *Lifestyle factors, cardiovascular disease and all-cause mortality in middle-aged and elderly women: a systematic review and meta-analysis.* Eur J Epidemiol, 2018. **33**(9): p. 831-845.

492. El Khoudary, S.R., et al., *Menopause Transition and Cardiovascular Disease Risk: Implications for Timing of Early Prevention: A Scientific Statement From the American Heart Association.* Circulation, 2020. **142**(25): p. e506-e532.

493. Ponnampalam, E.N., N.J. Mann, and A.J. Sinclair, *Effect of feeding systems on*

omega-3 fatty acids, conjugated linoleic acid and trans fatty acids in Australian beef cuts: potential impact on human health. Asia Pac J Clin Nutr, 2006. **15**(1): p. 21-9.

494. Sinclair, A., et al., *The ω-3 fatty acid content of canned, smoked and fresh fish in Australia.* 1998.

495. Rissanen, T., et al., *Fish oil-derived fatty acids, docosahexaenoic acid and docosapentaenoic acid, and the risk of acute coronary events: the Kuopio ischaemic heart disease risk factor study.* Circulation, 2000. **102**(22): p. 2677-9.

496. Akiba, S., et al., *Involvement of lipoxygenase pathway in docosapentaenoic acid-induced inhibition of platelet aggregation.* Biol Pharm Bull, 2000. **23**(11): p. 1293-7.

497. Semenov, M.V., et al., *Does fresh farmyard manure introduce surviving microbes into soil or activate soil-borne microbiota?* J Environ Manage, 2021. **294**: p. 113018.

498. Brothers, R.M., P.J. Fadel, and D.M. Keller, *Racial disparities in cardiovascular disease risk: mechanisms of vascular dysfunction.* Am J Physiol Heart Circ Physiol, 2019. **317**(4): p. H777-h789.

499. Agostino, J.W., et al., *Cardiovascular disease risk assessment for Aboriginal and Torres Strait Islander adults aged under 35 years: a consensus statement.* Med J Aust, 2020. **212**(9): p. 422-427.

500. Melisko, M.E., et al., *Vaginal Testosterone Cream vs Estradiol Vaginal Ring for Vaginal Dryness or Decreased Libido in Women Receiving Aromatase Inhibitors for Early-Stage Breast Cancer: A Randomized Clinical Trial.* JAMA Oncol, 2017. **3**(3): p. 313-319.

501. Islam, R.M., et al., *Safety and efficacy of testosterone for women: a systematic review and meta-analysis of randomised controlled trial data.* Lancet Diabetes Endocrinol, 2019. **7**(10): p. 754-766.

502. Reed, B.G., L. Bou Nemer, and B.R. Carr, *Has testosterone passed the test in premenopausal women with low libido? A systematic review.* Int J Womens Health, 2016. **8**: p. 599-607.

503. Labrie, F., et al., *Effect of intravaginal dehydroepiandrosterone (Prasterone) on libido and sexual dysfunction in postmenopausal women.* Menopause, 2009. **16**(5): p. 923-31.

504. Abedi, P., et al., *The Impact of Oxytocin Vaginal Gel on Sexual Function in Postmenopausal Women: A Randomized Controlled Trial.* J Sex Marital Ther, 2020. **46**(4): p. 377-384.

505. Diamond, L.E., et al., *Double-blind, placebo-controlled evaluation of the safety, pharmacokinetic properties and pharmacodynamic effects of intranasal PT-141, a melanocortin receptor agonist, in healthy males and patients with mild-to-moderate erectile dysfunction.* Int J Impot Res, 2004. **16**(1): p. 51-9.

506. Simon, J.A., et al., *Long-Term Safety and Efficacy of Bremelanotide for Hypoactive Sexual Desire Disorder.* Obstet Gynecol, 2019. **134**(5): p. 909-917.

507. Dunietz, G.L., et al., *Oxytocin and women's health in midlife.* J Endocrinol, 2024. **262**(1).

508. Gibon, E., L. Lu, and S.B. Goodman, *Aging, inflammation, stem cells, and bone healing.* Stem Cell Res Ther, 2016. **7**: p. 44.
509. Adamopoulos, I.E., *Inflammation in bone physiology and pathology.* Curr Opin Rheumatol, 2018. **30**(1): p. 59-64.
510. Athimulam, S., et al., *The Impact of Mild Autonomous Cortisol Secretion on Bone Turnover Markers.* J Clin Endocrinol Metab, 2020. **105**(5): p. 1469-77.
511. Piovezan, J.M., M.O. Premaor, and F.V. Comim, *Negative impact of polycystic ovary syndrome on bone health: a systematic review and meta-analysis.* Hum Reprod Update, 2019. **25**(5): p. 633-645.
512. Shams-White, M.M., et al., *Animal versus plant protein and adult bone health: A systematic review and meta-analysis from the National Osteoporosis Foundation.* PLoS One, 2018. **13**(2): p. e0192459.
513. Zhao, R., M. Zhang, and Q. Zhang, *The Effectiveness of Combined Exercise Interventions for Preventing Postmenopausal Bone Loss: A Systematic Review and Meta-analysis.* J Orthop Sports Phys Ther, 2017. **47**(4): p. 241-251.
514. Sanudo, B., et al., *A systematic review of the exercise effect on bone health: the importance of assessing mechanical loading in perimenopausal and postmenopausal women.* Menopause, 2017. **24**(10): p. 1208-1216.
515. Cava, E., N.C. Yeat, and B. Mittendorfer, *Preserving Healthy Muscle during Weight Loss.* Adv Nutr, 2017. **8**(3): p. 511-519.
516. Verreijen, A.M., et al., *A high whey protein-, leucine-, and vitamin D-enriched supplement preserves muscle mass during intentional weight loss in obese older adults: a double-blind randomized controlled trial.* Am J Clin Nutr, 2015. **101**(2): p. 279-86.
517. Wang, Y., et al., *Tai Chi Exercise for the Quality of Life in a Perimenopausal Women Organization: A Systematic Review.* Worldviews Evid Based Nurs, 2017. **14**(4): p. 294-305.
518. Papadopoulou, S.K., *Sarcopenia: A Contemporary Health Problem among Older Adult Populations.* Nutrients, 2020. **12**(5).
519. Cruz-Jentoft, A.J., et al., *Sarcopenia: revised European consensus on definition and diagnosis.* Age Ageing, 2019. **48**(1): p. 16-31.
520. Bergquist, R., et al., *Muscle Activity in Upper-Body Single-Joint Resistance Exercises with Elastic Resistance Bands vs. Free Weights.* J Hum Kinet, 2018. **61**: p. 5-13.
521. Baker, B.S., et al., *Does Blood Flow Restriction Therapy in Patients Older Than Age 50 Result in Muscle Hypertrophy, Increased Strength, or Greater Physical Function? A Systematic Review.* Clin Orthop Relat Res, 2020. **478**(3): p. 593-606.
522. Jønsson, A.B., et al., *Feasibility and estimated efficacy of blood flow restricted training in female patients with rheumatoid arthritis: a randomized controlled pilot study.* Scand J Rheumatol, 2021. **50**(3): p. 169-177.
523. Nascimento, D.D.C., et al., *A Useful Blood Flow Restriction Training Risk Stratification for Exercise and Rehabilitation.* Front Physiol, 2022. **13**: p. 808622.
524. Chiodini, I. and M.J. Bolland, *Calcium supplementation in osteoporosis: useful or harmful?* Eur J Endocrinol, 2018. **178**(4): p. D13-d25.

525. Mandatori, D., et al., *The Dual Role of Vitamin K2 in "Bone-Vascular Crosstalk": Opposite Effects on Bone Loss and Vascular Calcification.* Nutrients, 2021. **13**(4).
526. Rondanelli, M., et al., *Pivotal role of boron supplementation on bone health: A narrative review.* J Trace Elem Med Biol, 2020. **62**: p. 126577.
527. Gil, Á., J. Plaza-Diaz, and M.D. Mesa, *Vitamin D: Classic and Novel Actions.* Ann Nutr Metab, 2018. **72**(2): p. 87-95.
528. Ma, M.L., et al., *Efficacy of vitamin K2 in the prevention and treatment of postmenopausal osteoporosis: A systematic review and meta-analysis of randomized controlled trials.* Front Public Health, 2022. **10**: p. 979649.
529. Hasific, S., et al., *Effects of vitamins K2 and D3 supplementation in patients with severe coronary artery calcification: a study protocol for a randomised controlled trial.* BMJ Open, 2023. **13**(7): p. e073233.
530. Knapen, M.H., et al., *Three-year low-dose menaquinone-7 supplementation helps decrease bone loss in healthy postmenopausal women.* Osteoporos Int, 2013. **24**(9): p. 2499-507.
531. Theuwissen, E., et al., *Effect of low-dose supplements of menaquinone-7 (vitamin K2) on the stability of oral anticoagulant treatment: dose-response relationship in healthy volunteers.* J Thromb Haemost, 2013. **11**(6): p. 1085-92.
532. Khaliq, H., Z. Juming, and P. Ke-Mei, *The Physiological Role of Boron on Health.* Biol Trace Elem Res, 2018. **186**(1): p. 31-51.
533. James, G.P., *Dietary Boron, Brain Function, and Cognitive Performance.* Environmental health perspectives, 1994. **102**(7): p. 65-72.
534. Litovitz, T.L., et al., *Clinical manifestations of toxicity in a series of 784 boric acid ingestions.* Am J Emerg Med, 1988. **6**(3): p. 209-13.
535. Maria, S., et al., *Melatonin-micronutrients Osteopenia Treatment Study (MOTS): a translational study assessing melatonin, strontium (citrate), vitamin D3 and vitamin K2 (MK7) on bone density, bone marker turnover and health related quality of life in postmenopausal osteopenic women following a one-year double-blind RCT and on osteoblast-osteoclast co-cultures.* Aging (Albany NY), 2017. **9**(1): p. 256-285.
536. Popova, E.V., et al., *Boron - A potential goiterogen?* Med Hypotheses, 2017. **104**: p. 63-67.
537. Wright, F. and R.B. Weller, *Risks and benefits of UV radiation in older people: More of a friend than a foe?* Maturitas, 2015. **81**(4): p. 425-31.
538. Matta, M.K., et al., *Effect of Sunscreen Application Under Maximal Use Conditions on Plasma Concentration of Sunscreen Active Ingredients: A Randomized Clinical Trial.* Jama, 2019. **321**(21): p. 2082-2091.
539. Santoro, N., C.N. Epperson, and S.B. Mathews, *Menopausal Symptoms and Their Management.* Endocrinol Metab Clin North Am, 2015. **44**(3): p. 497-515.
540. Malik, R. and P. Meghana Reddy, *Effectiveness of Tibolone in Relieving Postmenopausal Symptoms for a Short-Term Period in Indian Women.* J Obstet Gynaecol India, 2023. **73**(3): p. 242-247.

541. Castrejón-Delgado, L., et al., *Effect of Tibolone on Bone Mineral Density in Post-menopausal Women: Systematic Review and Meta-Analysis.* Biology (Basel), 2021. **10**(3).

542. Kim, H.K., et al., *Comparison of the Efficacy of Tibolone and Transdermal Estrogen in Treating Menopausal Symptoms in Postmenopausal Women.* J Menopausal Med, 2019. **25**(3): p. 123-129.

543. Lello, S., et al., *Tibolone and Breast Tissue: a Review.* Reprod Sci, 2023. **30**(12): p. 3403-3409.

544. Henneicke-von Zepelin, H.H., *60 years of Cimicifuga racemosa medicinal products : Clinical research milestones, current study findings and current development.* Wien Med Wochenschr, 2017. **167**(7-8): p. 147-159.

545. Myers, S.P. and V. Vigar, *Effects of a standardised extract of Trifolium pratense (Promensil) at a dosage of 80mg in the treatment of menopausal hot flushes: A systematic review and meta-analysis.* Phytomedicine, 2017. **24**: p. 141-147.

546. Hitchcock, C.L. and J.C. Prior, *Oral micronized progesterone for vasomotor symptoms--a placebo-controlled randomized trial in healthy postmenopausal women.* Menopause, 2012. **19**(8): p. 886-93.

547. Gompel, A. and G. Plu-Bureau, *Progesterone, progestins and the breast in menopause treatment.* Climacteric, 2018. **21**(4): p. 326-332.

548. Yuk, J.S., *Relationship between menopausal hormone therapy and breast cancer: A nationwide population-based cohort study.* Int J Gynaecol Obstet, 2024.

549. Chlebowski, R.T., et al., *Association of Menopausal Hormone Therapy With Breast Cancer Incidence and Mortality During Long-term Follow-up of the Women's Health Initiative Randomized Clinical Trials.* Jama, 2020. **324**(4): p. 369-380.

550. Mittal, M., et al., *Impact of micronised progesterone and medroxyprogesterone acetate in combination with transdermal oestradiol on cardiovascular markers in women diagnosed with premature ovarian insufficiency or an early menopause: a randomised pilot trial.* Maturitas, 2022. **161**: p. 18-26.

551. Graham, S., et al., *Review of menopausal hormone therapy with estradiol and proges-terone versus other estrogens and progestins.* Gynecol Endocrinol, 2022. **38**(11): p. 891-910.

552. Trabert, B., et al., *Progesterone and Breast Cancer.* Endocr Rev, 2020. **41**(2): p. 320-44.

553. Fournier, A., F. Berrino, and F. Clavel-Chapelon, *Unequal risks for breast cancer associated with different hormone replacement therapies: results from the E3N cohort study.* Breast Cancer Res Treat, 2008. **107**(1): p. 103-11.

554. Støer, N.C., et al., *Menopausal hormone therapy and breast cancer risk: a population-based cohort study of 1.3 million women in Norway.* Br J Cancer, 2024. **131**(1): p. 126-137.

555. Yuk, J.S., et al., *Breast cancer risk association with postmenopausal hormone therapy: Health Insurance Database in South Korea-based cohort study.* Eur J Endocrinol, 2024. **190**(1): p. 1-11.

556. Cheng, J., et al., *The origin and evolution of the diosgenin biosynthetic pathway in yam.* Plant Commun, 2021. **2**(1): p. 100079.

557. Fabian, C.J., et al., *Effect of Bazedoxifene and Conjugated Estrogen (Duavee) on Breast Cancer Risk Biomarkers in High-Risk Women: A Pilot Study.* Cancer Prev Res (Phila), 2019. **12**(10): p. 711-720.

558. Bhupathiraju, S.N., et al., *Hormone Therapy Use and Risk of Chronic Disease in the Nurses' Health Study: A Comparative Analysis With the Women's Health Initiative.* Am J Epidemiol, 2017. **186**(6): p. 696-708.

559. Thompson, J.J., C. Ritenbaugh, and M. Nichter, *Why women choose compounded bioidentical hormone therapy: lessons from a qualitative study of menopausal decision-making.* BMC Womens Health, 2017. **17**(1): p. 97.

560. Trenor, C.C., 3rd, et al., *Hormonal contraception and thrombotic risk: a multidisciplinary approach.* Pediatrics, 2011. **127**(2): p. 347-57.

561. Bezwada, P., A. Shaikh, and D. Misra, *The Effect of Transdermal Estrogen Patch Use on Cardiovascular Outcomes: A Systematic Review.* J Womens Health (Larchmt), 2017. **26**(12): p. 1319-1325.

562. Files, J. and J.M. Kling, *Transdermal delivery of bioidentical estrogen in menopausal hormone therapy: a clinical review.* Expert Opin Drug Deliv, 2020. **17**(4): p. 543-549.

563. Yi, T., et al., *Transdermal estrogen gel vs oral estrogen after hysteroscopy for intrauterine adhesion separation: A prospective randomized study.* Front Endocrinol (Lausanne), 2023. **14**: p. 1066210.

564. Newman, M.S., et al., *Assessment of estrogen exposure from transdermal estradiol gel therapy with a dried urine assay.* Steroids, 2022. **184**: p. 109038.

565. Hipolito Rodrigues, M.A. and A. Gompel, *Micronized progesterone, progestins, and menopause hormone therapy.* Women Health, 2021. **61**(1): p. 3-14.

566. Backstrom, T., et al., *Paradoxical effects of GABA-A modulators may explain sex steroid induced negative mood symptoms in some persons.* Neuroscience, 2011. **191**: p. 46-54.

567. Labrie, F., et al., *Efficacy of intravaginal dehydroepiandrosterone (DHEA) on moderate to severe dyspareunia and vaginal dryness, symptoms of vulvovaginal atrophy, and of the genitourinary syndrome of menopause.* Menopause, 2018. **25**(11): p. 1339-1353.

568. Barton, D.L., et al., *Evaluating the efficacy of vaginal dehydroepiandosterone for vaginal symptoms in postmenopausal cancer survivors: NCCTG N10C1 (Alliance).* Support Care Cancer, 2018. **26**(2): p. 643-650.

569. Clabaut, M., et al., *Effect of 17β-estradiol on a human vaginal Lactobacillus crispatus strain.* Sci Rep, 2021. **11**(1): p. 7133.

570. Mueck, A.O., et al., *Treatment of vaginal atrophy with estriol and lactobacilli combination: a clinical review.* Climacteric, 2018. **21**(2): p. 140-147.

571. Chee, W.J.Y., S.Y. Chew, and L.T.L. Than, *Vaginal microbiota and the potential of*

Lactobacillus derivatives in maintaining vaginal health. Microb Cell Fact, 2020. **19**(1): p. 203.

572. Ali, E.S., C. Mangold, and A.N. Peiris, *Estriol: emerging clinical benefits.* Menopause, 2017. **24**(9): p. 1081-1085.

573. Farrell, R., *ACOG Committee Opinion No. 659: The Use of Vaginal Estrogen in Women With a History of Estrogen-Dependent Breast Cancer.* Obstet Gynecol, 2016. **127**(3): p. e93-6.

574. Hirschberg, A.L., et al., *Efficacy and safety of ultra-low dose 0.005% estriol vaginal gel for the treatment of vulvovaginal atrophy in postmenopausal women with early breast cancer treated with nonsteroidal aromatase inhibitors: a phase II, randomized, double-blind, placebo-controlled trial.* Menopause, 2020. **27**(5): p. 526-534.

575. McVicker, L., et al., *Vaginal Estrogen Therapy Use and Survival in Females With Breast Cancer.* JAMA Oncol, 2024. **10**(1): p. 103-108.

576. Cardone, A., et al., *Utilisation of hydrogen peroxide in the treatment of recurrent bacterial vaginosis.* Minerva Ginecol, 2003. **55**(6): p. 483-92.

577. Powell, A., et al., *Clinicians' Use of Intravaginal Boric Acid Maintenance Therapy for Recurrent Vulvovaginal Candidiasis and Bacterial Vaginosis.* Sex Transm Dis, 2019. **46**(12): p. 810-812.

578. Sobel, R. and J.D. Sobel, *Metronidazole for the treatment of vaginal infections.* Expert Opin Pharmacother, 2015. **16**(7): p. 1109-15.

579. Genovese, C., et al., *Combined systemic (fluconazole) and topical (metronidazole + clotrimazole) therapy for a new approach to the treatment and prophylaxis of recurrent candidiasis.* Minerva Ginecol, 2019. **71**(4): p. 321-328.

580. Homayouni, A., et al., *Effects of probiotics on the recurrence of bacterial vaginosis: a review.* J Low Genit Tract Dis, 2014. **18**(1): p. 79-86.

581. Jeng, H.S., T.R. Yan, and J.Y. Chen, *Treating vaginitis with probiotics in non-pregnant females: A systematic review and meta-analysis.* Exp Ther Med, 2020. **20**(4): p. 3749-3765.

582. Abou Chacra, L., F. Fenollar, and K. Diop, *Bacterial Vaginosis: What Do We Currently Know?* Front Cell Infect Microbiol, 2021. **11**: p. 672429.

583. Ng, Q.X., et al., *Use of Lactobacillus spp. to prevent recurrent urinary tract infections in females.* Med Hypotheses, 2018. **114**: p. 49-54.

584. Harlow, S.D., et al., *Executive summary of the Stages of Reproductive Aging Workshop + 10: addressing the unfinished agenda of staging reproductive aging.* J Clin Endocrinol Metab, 2012. **97**(4): p. 1159-68.

www.ingramcontent.com/pod-product-compliance
Lightning Source LLC
Chambersburg PA
CBHW040828300326
41914CB00059B/1290